CNA CAREER LADDER MADE EASY

This book is dedicated to those who do the hardest, most important job in America — nursing assistants. Were it not for their commitment, compassion, and skill, our elders would be without the loving care they deserve. Angels of mercy, guardians, healers, heroes — they are a shining example to us all.

CNA CAREER LADDER MADE EASY

Everything You Need to Run a Successful Career Ladder Program

By Dr. Karl Pillemer, Rhoda Meador, Richard Hoffman, and Martin Schumacher

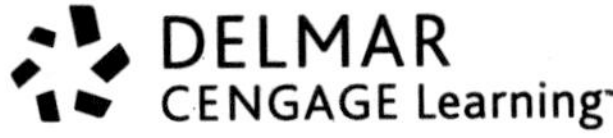

Australia • Brazil • Japan • Korea • Mexico • Singapore • Spain • United Kingdom • United States

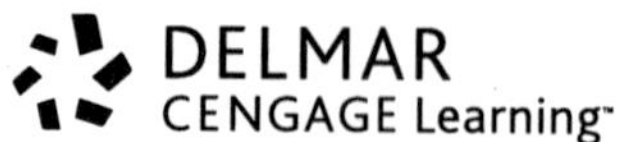

CNA Career Ladder Made Easy: EverythingYou Need to Run a Successful Career Ladder Program

Karl Pillemer, Rhoda Meador, Richard Hoffman, and Martin Schumacher

For product information and technology assistance, contact us at **Cengage Learning Customer & Sales Support, 1-800-354-9706**

For permission to use material from this text or product, submit all requests online at **www.cengage.com/permissions**
Further permissions questions can be emailed to **permissionrequest@cengage.com**

ISBN-13: 978-0-9653629-6-2

ISBN-10: 0-9653629-6-5

Delmar
Executive Woods
5 Maxwell Drive
Clifton Park, NY 12065
USA

Cengage Learning is a leading provider of customized learning solutions with office locations around the globe, including Singapore, the United Kingdom, Australia, Mexico, Brazil, and Japan. Locate your local office at **www.cengage.com/global**

Cengage Learning products are represented in Canada by Nelson Education, Ltd.

To learn more about Delmar, visit **www.cengage.com/delmar**

Purchase any of our products at your local bookstore or at our preferred online store **www.ichapters.com**

Printed in the United States of America
3 4 5 6 7 15 14 13 12 11

FD214

CONTENTS

ABOUT THE AUTHORS

Karl Pillemer

Karl Pillemer, Ph.D, is a Professor in the Human Development Department and Director of the Gerontology Research Institute at Cornell University. A consultant to major long-term care providers across the country, Dr. Pillemer has conducted research and developed practical programs to improve the work life of nursing home staff. He is also a founder and Executive Editor of Frontline Publishing.

Rhoda Meador

Rhoda Meador, MS, is the Director of Curriculum Development for Delmar, Cengage Learning. She has developed, field-tested, and implemented many successful long-term care staff training programs on topics including mentoring, elder abuse, and communications. Her administrative and research activities have centered on promoting greater understanding among staff in institutional settings. She is a frequent guest speaker at regional and national conferences.

Richard Hoffman

Richard Hoffman works closely with leading figures in all areas of healthcare to synthesize Delmar's ongoing content development. He has worked in healthcare administration for over a decade. In addition to being the voice of *Nursing Assistant Monthly,* Richard serves as a consultant to the industry press, and regularly publishes articles and speaks on the subject of professional development for Delmar caregivers.

Martin Schumacher

As one of Delmar's founders, Martin oversees the development and publication of its continuing education publications (*Nursing Assistant Monthly* and *The Resident Assistant*), its staff retention programs, and its many books for the healthcare industry. Prior to launching Delmar, Martin spent 15 years in print communications, developing educational and training programs for large companies and organizations.

Preface

The book you hold in your hand is based on years of work culling ideas from best practices throughout long-term care. It not only represents the state-of-the-art in career ladder programs, it is also designed to be extremely simple and easy to use. This straightforward and practical program will begin to improve your facility's CNA retention picture immediately, not to mention your staff's morale and the care your residents receive.

CNAs are often treated as if they are workers whose jobs require few skills. Nothing could be further from the truth! CNAs shoulder tremendous responsibilities. More than anyone else in a long-term care facility, they are responsible for the daily health and well-being of the residents. To meet this responsibility requires a complex set of technical, social, problem-solving and communication skills. In short, the kinds of skills required of a professional. Until now, however, few CNAs have been offered a profession. Instead of a career, they are generally offered a locked-in, no-growth job which almost ensures that they will eventually move on to something else. A career ladder program, on the other hand, offers them a sense of pride and feeling of professionalism in their position.

By implementing the program found in this book, you are investing in your CNAs. The program will offer your nursing assistants the skills, encouragement, and confidence that will help them develop into quality health care professionals. Implementing this program will not only help you train and reward your CNAs, it will also help knit them into a smoothly functioning caregiving team. If your facility invests the time and energy, this program will help you reduce your facility's CNA turnover, save you money, and build a more loyal staff.

This book, however, is nothing more than a set of tools. What you do with these tools will determine the effectiveness of the program. In fact, the single most important factor to the success of a career ladder program is, well, YOU. Our experience has shown us that programs that have had a "champion" — someone wholly committed to their success — have made a profound difference in a facility's morale, work-culture, quality of care, and rate of attrition. We have tried to make it as easy as possible for you, but it's up to you and your facility to make it all come together. This program will require your time and energy, as well as the support of the entire facility. For this program to have a lasting, positive effect, for this program to be the agent of genuine change in your organization, your whole facility must be committed to its success — from the administrator to the program's students.

In this first section, you will find instructions and recommendations on how to implement a successful career ladder program. Think of it as your owner's manual. Here we will lay out the program for you, starting with the big picture — why the program exists and what it will do for you. Then we give you guidelines on how to implement and administer the program — from selecting your students to rewarding your graduates. Finally, we spell out the specific steps you need to take to launch and run your program.

Implementing Your Career Ladder Program

As we begin a new century, CNAs will have an increasingly important position in the care of the elderly. As their importance increases, the necessity for training and empowering them increases. The irony in the long-term care industry is that we want career nursing assistants, but we don't offer them a career. For this reason, turnover is a major problem that affects not only a facility's finances, but the sense of morale and teamwork among staff.

A career ladder program offers one solution to the chronic problem of CNA turnover. It enhances CNAs' knowledge and skills, and provides them an opportunity for advancement. It creates a support system and sense of teamwork for nursing assistants. For the facility, making nursing assistants feel more professional leads to better quality care, increased employee morale, and reduced turnover. We designed the *CNA Career Ladder Made Easy* to be a complete, ready-to-use program, with everything your facility needs right here in one book.

Goals of a CNA Career Ladder Program

Why invest time and energy in a career ladder program? Experts say there are a number of good reasons. Here are a few of them:

- To enhance the professional knowledge and skills of CNAs.
- To provide CNAs with a genuine opportunity for advancement in their facility.
- To boost CNAs' sense of self-worth and commitment to their job.
- And, ultimately, to improve resident care and to reduce CNA turnover.

Who is Eligible?

Your facility will need to establish the eligibility requirements for students to be considered for your career ladder program. As a baseline, we recommend that each applicant:

- Be a Certified Nursing Assistant (CNA).
- Be state certified.
- Meet your facility's hiring criteria.

We also recommend that you establish additional requirements to ensure that only those individuals who are serious about the program and about their future in long-term care apply. Not every CNA will be suited to this program; that needs to be made clear from the start. You will set your own additional standards for acceptance into the program, but we suggest the following:

- Successful completion of your facility's orientation program.
- Completion of six (6) months continuous service with a satisfactory attendance record.
- Satisfactory performance evaluations.
- No disciplinary action in the past six (6) months.

Promoting the Program

Your CNAs will need to know about the program, what it is, and why it's important to them. Have your DON or staff development coordinator talk to those CNAs who they think would be good candidates. Announce the program at your next all-staff or CNA meeting, and let them know the eligibility requirements and how to go about applying. Make it clear who CNAs can go to with questions and who will be handling the application process.

Application Process

To apply for the career ladder program, interested CNAs should fill out your facility application form (a sample is included in the back of this book). The form should require that they write a brief essay about why they want to participate in the program. The applicant should turn this form into their supervisor, or other designated individual, who will be responsible for determining the applicant's eligibility and for getting the form signed by your facility's DON and/or administrator.

Once applications have been submitted, your program planning group (see description below) should review all the applications, discuss each prospective student, and then inform, verbally or by written letter, the chosen participants. You should include congratulations, as well as instructions on class time and place. An informational meeting with the chosen students should be held by the class instructor before the class starts to talk about the expectations, requirements, and rewards for successful completion of the program. You should also contact those applicants who did not make it into the first class to thank them and encourage their future involvement in the program.

Program Curriculum

We've designed the curriculum in an easy-to-follow, scripted format so that you, the instructor, can, with little preparation, start running your class right away. We hope you find it a pleasure to use, and that you make it your own.

Each of the nine modules is designed to take three hours of classroom instruction. For your students to receive maximum benefit from this program, we recommend classes be scheduled in a concentrated period of time, preferably one module (or subject) per week for nine consecutive weeks.

Each of the program's nine modules follows the same format:

- In the beginning — goals of the module
- Introduction — for the instructor only
- The speaker's script (with instructions)
- Handouts (to be distributed to class participants)
- At the end — a quiz (for class participants).

In addition, scattered throughout each module are group exercises and activities — like role-playing, word games, and brainstorming — to help make each session an enjoyable and memorable learning experience for your CNAs. Plan to use a classroom or designated area where you won't be interrupted and your class can be comfortable and relaxed.

To make the teaching process easy for you, each module is written in a script format that includes the following icons to indicate specific activities for the instructor:

SAY the following text to the class.

READ the following passage or handout to the class.

WRITE the following words for the whole class to see.

DISTRIBUTE the following handout or quiz to the class.

STOP TAKE A BREAK offers an opportunity for the class to take a break.

A HOT IDEA is a different or fun idea for a class exercise.

Note: Text that is intended only for the instructor appears in italic form and has no icon connected to it.

Once you start using these modules, we trust that you'll find this scripted format very easy to use.

How the Curriculum Is Organized

The Career Ladder curriculum in this book consists of nine (9) modules of classroom training to be completed in twenty-seven (27) hours. Each training module is listed below along with its time-frame and content objectives.

Module 1 — Safety First (3 hours)

CNAs will:

- Learn infection control techniques
- Review fire and emergency procedures
- Explore ways of reducing resident falls
- Master safe transfers

Module 2 — Teamwork and Cooperation (3 hours)

CNAs will:

- Achieve a greater understanding of the concept of teamwork and how an effective team functions
- See their central role in good caregiving
- Explore the benefits and responsibilities of teamwork, especially as it relates to staff from other departments
- Learn about the other departments' functions and responsibilities

Module 3 — Aging and Illness (3 hours)

CNAs will:

- Understand the physical and functional changes that accompany normal aging, and learn to distinguish these from the symptoms of disease
- Understand three diseases commonly found in older people and learn measures to address problems associated with them

Module 4 — Communication is Key (3 hours)

CNAs will:

- Learn specific tactics for improving communication
- Discover the importance of clear communication in the facility
- Learn to identify possible impediments to open, productive communication

Module 5 — Nutrition (3 hours)

CNAs will:

- Learn the basics of good nutrition and hydration for older adults
- Be alert to the warning signs of nutritional problems and the conditions of nutritional risk
- Learn factors that affect eating ability and appetite

Module 6 — Spirituality and Dying (3 hours)

CNAs will:

- Learn to ease the fears and anxieties and that can go along with death in a nursing facility
- Appreciate residents' different spiritual needs so they can offer emotional support and understanding
- Learn the importance of mourning when a beloved resident dies

Module 7 — Your Residents' Quality of Life (3 hours)

CNAs will:

- Outline ways to make new residents feel at home
- Learn the need to understand and empathize with their residents
- Foster the residents' independence while committing to a defense of their rights
- Be alert to the signs of psychosocial difficulties, especially depression

Module 8 — Dementia Care (3 hours)

CNAs will:

- Outline the fundamentals of what constitutes dementia
- Learn a practical approach for handling problem behaviors associated with dementia
- Look at difficult behaviors as a form of communication

Module 9 — The Importance of Family (3 hours)

CNAs will:

- Learn that they must work together with family members to achieve the best care for the resident
- Gain new insight into family members' occasionally frustrating behavior
- Be empowered to act calmly and professionally in stressful situations with residents' families

How to Get Started

Once the students have been selected for your first class, a classroom chosen, and a schedule established, it's time to prepare for your first class. While the program has been designed for quick implementation, there are three simple steps you need to take:

1. Review your first module or unit of instruction, including the related handouts. The lectures contained in each module are meant to convey basic knowledge and information of a topic. They are not meant to be read word for word. Your should familiarize yourself with the content, then feel free to make it your own. Most pages in the Instructor's Guidebook have room on which to write speaker notes. One simple way to personalize your lectures is to add examples and names from your own facility.
2. Check to see if the content calls for any special resource or outside representative to be included. A few of the modules do require a little extra preparation prior to your class instruction, such as gathering a few materials or inviting a facility representative to make a presentation.
3. Make enough photocopies of the handouts (including the quiz) for each class participant. Do not plan to distribute the handouts until your script calls for it. The handouts are an effective learning tool that reinforce the lectures in each module.

At the end of each classroom session or module your students should take the basic true/false quiz provided. This quiz is not the method to evaluate whether a student passes or not. It simply offers them a chance to review the major points of each module, while giving you a means to measure their progress. Answers to the quiz are found at the end of each module. Each class should conclude with you collecting the completed quizzes to keep in each student's file.

If you can, plan to give each of your class participants a binder at the start of the program so they can collect the handouts throughout the course. These handouts, gathered together, will serve as review text for your students. As another tool for classroom instruction, you might consider copying some or all of these handouts onto acetate to project as transparencies.

A Final Note

Every instructor has his or her own teaching style. Whatever yours may be, make sure you involve every one of your students in the class. Do whatever you can to make them feel comfortable yet focused. Encourage them to participate. Engage them mentally as well as emotionally, get them laughing — and wonderful things will happen. Good luck!

Class Structure and Scheduling

We recommend classes take place in your facility once a week for nine weeks. Each module should take up to, but not exceed, three hours, allowing for a 15-minute break somewhere in the middle (we recommend a natural break in each module, but feel free to set your own pace). Class time should be set to suit the majority of people's schedules or, if you can, arrange with your facility to make the students' work schedules suit your class time. Many facilities find that evening classes are the easiest to accommodate everyone's schedule.

Lecturing is kept to a minimum and is interspersed with class exercises, role-plays, case studies, and handouts to review and write on. There is no time limit for the exercises or the review of the handouts; set times at your discretion. It should depend on how many students are involved and on the class's enthusiasm for that particular activity. At the end of each class period, the quiz should be distributed and ample time allowed for students to complete it. The instructor should keep all completed quizzes on file.

Your class size should be small, between nine and twelve students. A small class size makes it possible to create a level of comfort and intimacy impossible with a larger group, while allowing everyone to participate regularly.

Class setting is as integral to the student's comfort as class size. For time and financial reasons, you will probably want to conduct it within your facility. Find a room with enough space where the students can move around and engage in the class exercises. Also, make sure to schedule the class in a place where residents or other staff will not interrupt.

Here are two final points regarding your Career Ladder program class:

1. We strongly recommend that your students get paid while they are in class. It is critical that your students understand that their facility is investing in them and in their future.
2. This program should not replace or alter, in any way, your facility's ongoing CNA in-service program.

Student Evaluations

To determine whether a student has successfully completed the program, we recommend the use of a pass/fail system. This is not to suggest that this program be taken lightly by the students or anyone else. On the contrary, we strongly recommend that specific guidelines for passing or failing the program be developed and made clear to all prospective students prior to the first class. Students should realize from the outset that this program is a serious undertaking, and no one will get a "free ride." The guidelines you establish for your pass/fail system should be based on the following factors:

- **Class participation.** Was the student an active participant? Did he or she contribute to the group exercises and ask thoughtful questions? Even if a student was less talkative, did you sense that he or she was engaged and taking the class activities seriously?

- **Attendance.** We recommend 100 percent attendance as a requirement for all students. You may choose to offer make-up classes for students with viable excuses for missing a class. If any classes are missed and not made up, the student should understand that this constitutes voluntary withdrawal from the program.
- **Completed homework.** There are only a few instances of "homework" outside of the class. Any student who doesn't complete all of his or her assignments within a reasonable time should not receive a passing grade.
- **Quizzes.** We recommend student scores be at least 70 percent or above for all quizzes. Because we feel a student's pass/fail status should not rest on test scores, we recommend make-up quizzes be made available for those students who are genuinely trying, but may have trouble grasping a particular subject.

The instructor should keep a file for each student, recording all pertinent information affecting the student's pass/fail status, including all completed quizzes and homework. You may want to give a copy of the individual evaluations to each student and keep one on file in the facility for future reference.

Compensation and Rewards

What sort of financial compensation you give to your program's graduates is one of the most significant decisions your facility will make. Regarding this matter, we feel strongly: you should give a pay increase to each student that successfully completes the program. By doing so, you tell all of your staff that you recognize and appreciate the accomplishment of your program's graduates. Moreover, we strongly recommend that this pay increase be a significant amount, not less than a dollar an hour increase.

If, however, after serious consideration, your facility decides it can't offer such a pay increase, we then recommend you give out a one-time cash bonus to each graduate. And, similar to the pay increase, we strongly recommend that you make this bonus to be a significant amount of money. We recommend a minimum bonus of $250 per graduate.

Anything short of a significant pay increase or cash bonus will undercut the seriousness and credibility of your entire program. Whatever your facility decides, the specifics should be openly shared with all of your CNAs from the outset.

Recognition for Success

After the successful completion of the program, your facility should plan a graduation ceremony where all of your program's graduates are recognized and honored. Plan to make it a serious yet celebratory occasion where you hand out a diploma or special certificate (a sample is provided) to each graduate. And with the diploma or certificate, consider giving your graduates a new job title as well; possibilities might include "CNA II" or "Advanced Caregiver." Try to have your administrator and other department heads present, as well as other staff. In addition, have your graduates invite family and friends to attend. If possible, try to get a special speaker, such as the town's mayor or another prominent community figure to speak during the ceremony. Make it special. Make it a big deal. It will pay off for your CNAs and your facility.

In addition to your graduation ceremony, you may choose to recognize your graduates with special name tags or pins to designate their new status. Whatever you choose, make sure your graduates are clearly recognized for their hard work and commitment.

Six Easy Steps for Launching Your Program

Now that you are familiar with the primary issues involved in implementing a career ladder program, it's time to get started. Though every facility will launch and run this program in their own way, here is an outline of the major steps you should take to get your program up and running:

Step 1: Create a Career Ladder Planning Group

Organize a small group from your facility that will be committed to making sure the program gets properly launched and sustained. This group's mission will be to make the critical decisions that will shape the program in a way that best suits your CNAs and your facility. This group should include your administrator, your director of nursing, one or two experienced nursing assistants, and several other key members of your facility.

You need a good cross representation of your facility for two reasons. First, such a group represents a facility-wide commitment to foster CNA development and professionalism; other staff see that there is serious "buy-in" to the program. Secondly, the administration must be in on the ground floor for all decisions, such as pay increases and additional CNA hours, that will affect the facility's bottom-line.

The role of the planning group is to:

- Make all the key decisions regarding how the program will work: eligibility, the application and selection process, compensation and rewards, and all other major program logistics.
- Familiarize itself with the program by reviewing the entire curriculum and discussing ways to customize it.
- Select the program's instructor, and, with this individual, determine location and time for the classes.
- Evaluate all students' applications and choose who will participate.
- Monitor the program's progress and adjust accordingly.

Step 2: Make the Tough Decisions

Your planning group needs to determine how the program will specifically work within your facility. What policies and procedures will you establish? Using the appropriate sections of this document as your guide, your group should use the following questions and suggestions to start:

1. What are our eligibility requirements for entrance into the program?
2. How do we announce and promote the program to our CNAs and other staff?
3. What do we need on the application form specific to our facility? Who will be in charge of the application process?
4. What is the specific criteria for determining student success or failure in the program? How will this be communicated?
5. What will students who graduate from the program receive? What kind of pay increase or bonus can the facility commit to?
6. How will we recognize and honor our graduates? Who will be in charge of organizing a graduation ceremony?

Step 3: Choose Your Instructor

The group's next major task is to choose the primary instructor to run the classes. The first thing to do is review the curriculum closely, and then ask: who would be the best choice to conduct this training? Is it your staff development coordinator or is there someone else who might be better equipped? Your selection here is very important, as the instructor's approach and comfort level with the CNAs will have a major impact on the success of the program.

The curriculum is designed to engage the students emotionally, as well as intellectually. Most members of your first class will have been out of an academic setting for a long time or did not do well in school in the first place. To keep them engaged, the lectures are balanced with activities and involvement. There is a lot of difficult material to get through, but a confident and energetic teacher should be able to keep most of his or her students focused.

(Note: The authors strongly suggest you consider using an additional instructor or team of instructors to present certain topics or modules, such as safety or dementia care, that require specific knowledge. Where appropriate, instructions are provided at the beginning of some of the modules.)

Step 4: Prepare the Training

Preparation and rehearsal are key to a successful program. The more familiar your instructor is with the material, the better the class experience will be. If possible, the planning group might take part in a "dry run" of part of a module, so the instructor can have a chance to practice and the other planning members will get a better idea of what a class will be all about. The instructor should give some thought to his or her teaching style and how he or she is going to customize the program to the facility.

The instructor should also scan over all the modules, at least the beginning section of each, to see where additional participants and/or resources are called for. Finally, as a minimum, prior to teaching any of the modules, your instructor should scan over all the text for that unit, as well as closely read the instructor's introduction (i.e., "Introduction — For Instructor Only").

Step 5: Evaluate and Select Your Students

Once you've announced the program and received completed application forms, your group will need to evaluate and select the members of your first class. Again, each facility will be a little different, but you need to develop a clear procedure for your selection process. If you are swamped with eligible applicants — first, congratulate yourself, that's a good sign! — you will need to respond. Is it possible, given your resources, to schedule and run an additional class? If not, then plan to include those eligible students in another class later on in the year. Ideally, no one will be left out and your program will be available, at some point in time, to all interested and qualified CNAs.

Step 6: Determine Class Logistics

As previously mentioned, we recommend scheduling your class in a concentrated way, ideally once a week for a three-hour session for nine weeks. This deliberately "intensive" approach helps to create good group cohesion (a "we're all in this together" feeling) and a strong learning environment.

Holding your classes in-house will probably be most easy and cost-effective, but if you don't have a good, private location in your facility, consider an out-of-facility site where your students might feel more confident and open to new ideas.

Whatever location you choose, make sure it allows for privacy and comfort for all. And, whatever time you schedule for your class, make sure everyone can commit to it.

Launching and Running Your Career Ladder Program

SAMPLE TIMELINE — 14-WEEK PERIOD

1 2 3 4 5 6 7 8 9 10 11 12 13 14

WEEK 1 — Read *CNA Career Ladder Made Easy.*

WEEKS 2 - 14 — Promote the program on an ongoing basis.
Explain to facility stakeholders what a career ladder is and why it's important.

WEEKS 2, 3 — Choose your training instructor.

WEEKS 3, 4 — Recruit and select your trainees.
Determine eligibility requirements and solicit applications.

WEEKS 3, 4 — Determine class logistics.

WEEKS 5 - 13 — Conduct training classes:
teach one module per week, for nine consecutive weeks.

WEEKS 12, 13, 14 — Plan and execute a "graduation" to take place shortly after the training classes are completed.

Teaching and Learning

Understanding Adult Learning Styles

People learn in different ways. By the time we are adults we have developed certain ways of learning that we find work best for us. Whether you are in the role of learner or teacher, it is helpful to know your own learning style.

Most adults use a combination of learning styles, but each of us finds one of the following styles most comfortable:

1. The *visual* learner might say, "Show me. I'll watch. Then I'll know how." Keyword: EYES.
2. The *auditory* learner prefers to hear instructions. "If you explain it to me clearly, then I'll know how to do it." Keyword: EARS.
3. The *cognitive* or thinking learner might say something like, "Give me written directions. Let me study it, and I'll learn it." Keyword: BRAIN.
4. The *kinesthetic* or doing learner prefers trial and error. "Just let me do it over until I get it right. Then I'll know it." Keyword: HANDS.

In addition to learning style, a variety of other factors affect adult learning. Certain factors may be more critical to some people than to others.

- Level of interest of both the teacher and the learner
- Level of experience of the teacher
- Degree of preparation by the teacher
- Type of teaching methods
- Adequacy of teaching material
- Physical environment

- Emotional comfort level of both the teacher and the learner
- Levels of motivation of the both the teacher and the learner
- Maturity of the learner
- Health of the learner.

Creating a Learning Environment

Educators have learned that adults are motivated to learn when they understand the reason for what they are learning. As caregivers, your nursing assistants have the well-being of the residents, their physical, social, and emotional needs to motivate them. As employees, they now have opportunities for career growth within the company to motivate them to learn all they can about how to be the very best caregivers possible.

It is important for students and instructor together to take responsibility for creating a learning environment. In order to create an environment where people are sharing knowledge and information, there has to be respect for one another, an understanding of peoples' different ways of learning, and a great deal of patience. The rewards, however, are well worth it. Creating a learning environment means offering to help, demonstrating what you've learned to others, and making sure you give your students the support and encouragement they need. And it means continuing to be a committed learner yourself.

Generally speaking, nobody needs more negative criticism. One way to do this is to recognize the things your students do especially well, and ignore the things you think they might have done better. You will find that if you concentrate on the positive, you create an environment in which people can acknowledge their weaknesses and ask others for help. This is what we mean by a learning environment.

Understanding and Using Different Teaching Methods

When you were a child in school, you probably didn't think much about how your teachers were presenting the material; you focused completely on the content and did the best you could. As an adult, however, you have had enough experience to be aware of which teaching methods work best for you, and to be aware of your strengths and weaknesses as a learner. You may find it helpful to ask yourself, from time to time, which teaching method you are using and whether it matches the needs and learning styles of your students.

Teaching Methods

1. **Lecture**

   An organized oral presentation of material; useful for presenting factual information.

2. **Directed or Guided Discussion**

   Verbal exchange between two or more people; useful for problem solving and brainstorming.

3. **Demonstration**

   Presentation that shows how to perform a procedure; useful for skills training when a physical response from the learner is necessary.

4. **Hand-Over-Hand**

   Maneuvering of the learner's hand and arm; useful for skills training when a physical response from the learner is necessary.

5. Role Play

Simulates experiences and situations; useful for practicing skills and return demonstrations.

6. Peer Instruction

Allows learner to present experiences and material; useful for retaining learner's attention.

One of the most effective ways to learn something is to teach it to someone else by explaining or demonstrating it. From time to time you might ask participants to work in pairs or in a group. This can be a very powerful way to learn because students are bringing together the different learning styles, strengths, and capabilities of the group's members. Working together to be sure that everyone learns the material can be the most effective way for each individual member to be sure they have mastered it.

Effective learning includes continually reviewing and troubleshooting. Some experts recommend that adult learners keep a "learning journal." After each class or study session, have your students write a short, dated note to themselves in a notebook about how they think their learning is going. Remember that the idea is not for them to judge themselves, but to look honestly at what's working or not working in their learning process. A note in a learning journal might address the following questions:

- Do I understand the material?
- What do I think I need to do in order to master this new material?
- If I feel I need some help learning the material, whom can I ask? The instructor? A fellow student?
- What have I done to contribute to maintaining a "learning environment"?

Final Tips for Your Instructor

On a final note, before your first class begins, here are several suggestions we hope your instructor will take to heart:

DON'T — set your expectations too high in the beginning.

DON'T — be too rigid in following the curriculum. If an exercise or a role-play isn't working, move on to something else.

DON'T — read directly from the script. This is boring for both you and your class.

DON'T — forget about the importance of the training environment. Try to find a comfortable setting for your class and offer refreshments, if possible.

DON'T — assume that because a participant is quiet, that he or she is not learning anything; some people may have trouble speaking up, but are still learning.

DO — involve your administrator in the program from the very beginning, and keep him or her up-to-date on the progress.

DO — rehearse the exercises and role-plays before you teach the class.

DO — put the lectures in your own words.

DO — feel free to modify the case studies and role-plays to include situations that are more appropriate to your facility.

DO — set a relaxed and friendly tone in the classroom. This is not a place where people will be judged harshly; it is a group learning experience, where a participant's stories and experiences should play an integral part.

DO — have fun!

CNA
CAREER LADDER
MADE
EASY

Program Curriculum

MODULE 1

Safety First

Objectives of this Module

CNAs will:

- Learn infection control techniques
- Review fire and emergency procedures
- Explore ways of reducing resident falls
- Master safe transfers

Introduction

For Instructor Only

Everyone is at risk until no one is at risk. This must be the guiding rule in the hazardous world of nursing homes. And many of these dangers are invisible. Infection control, safe transfers, preventing falls, and fire/emergency procedures will be the main safety topics discussed in this first module.

TAKE NOTE: You should try to get representatives from other departments to address the class: someone on infection control, someone on emergency and fire safety, and a physical therapist for performing safe transfers. If they cannot visit the class, see if they can offer comments for you to deliver to the class.

TOPIC #1

Infection Control

To begin, SAY:

Infection control is the most important precaution a nursing home can take. Learning how to prevent and control infection will help you in protecting yourself, your residents, your fellow staff, and your resident's families. The first thing you need to understand is how infectious pathogens are spread, and then how to stop their spread.

Older adults can be fatally affected by infection; it is one of the leading causes of death for them. Knowing your facility's policies and procedures for infection control will help you build a barrier between your residents and the outside world. Infection control will also keep you healthier when dealing with seriously ill residents.

Someone need not be sick to be carrying a harmful pathogen that could make others sick. Since there is no way of telling who's carrying them, the best plan is to act as if they're potentially everywhere. This is why taking precautions is a key part of your job.

Protect yourself against infection a resident might be carrying. Wear gloves while handling a resident's blood, feces, urine, or mucous. Wash your hands before and after wearing the gloves. Report any sores on yourself or on a resident to your supervisor. Also, be aware that "sharps," like razor blades, needles, and knives, can all be infectious. Always wash up at the end of your shift to protect your family from infections you might be carrying.

Protect the resident from any infection you might be carrying. Wash up thoroughly at the beginning of your shift. Cover any cuts or sores with bandages. If you are not feeling well, coughing or sneezing, let your supervisor know. They can try to steer you away from residents who may be more susceptible to illness.

Washing up can be the simplest and most important thing you do to prevent the spread of infection. Though it may seem obvious, let's review the proper way to wash our hands. Remember, you should do this *before and after* you wear gloves, and many other times during your shift.

Show the class how to properly wash their hands. Have a class member distribute the first handout on handwashing, as you demonstrate proper technique. Also, be sure to point out bad handwashing habits, like washing without soap or drying them on your clothes.

DISTRIBUTE Handout 1-1: How to Wash Your Hands.

After reviewing the handout and demonstrating proper handwashing technique, ask your class what the most hazardous items in a facility are.

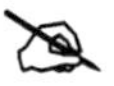

WRITE their responses on the board.

Then check to see if the following were listed. Discuss why each could be potentially harmful.

- *dentures*
- *toothbrushes*
- *hair brushes and combs*
- *razors*
- *needles*
- *silverware and cutlery*
- *horizontal surfaces, uncleaned*
- *bedpans and urinals*
- *soiled linen bins*
- *linen*
- *exposed food*
- *cups and glasses*

DISTRIBUTE Handout 1-2: Infection Control Terms.

After reviewing the handout, SAY:

Since antibiotic medications have become commonplace, some bacteria can resist usual medication. These kinds of infections (VRE and MRSA) may call for the resident to be isolated from other residents. It is essential that you protect yourself when dealing with a resident like this. Your supervisor should review infection control procedure with you, if you need to deal with an isolated patient.

TAKE NOTE: This would be a great place to have someone come speak about your facility's infection control procedures. If you are doing it yourself, make sure you clarify the following things:

- *What to do when accidentally exposed to biohazardous material.*
- *Whether to come to work and what precautions to take at work when you are feeling ill.*
- *How to handle infected, isolated residents.*
- *Getting influenza vaccines.*
- *Getting tested for TB.*
- *Disposing of contaminated medical waste.*

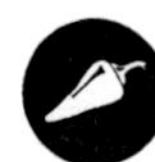

A Hot Idea

For a Class Exercise

This exercise will require preparation before class. Simulate each of the following in an empty room, then lead your class into the prepared room:

- Remove the infectious waste container from the room (or move it to an unsafe place)
- Fit one window with a torn screen
- Wet and "soil" the bed sheet
- Arrange bedclothes so they drag on the floor
- Place a toothbrush and hairbrush together on the nightstand
- Leave a jar of unwrapped candies open on the nightstand
- Remove paper towels from the bathroom
- Leave a syringe in the bathroom
- Put the toilet seat up

After your class inspects the room, ask them to list what possible infectious dangers lay in the room. Have them come up with a solution to each danger.

To continue, SAY:

The HIV/AIDS virus is becoming an enormous problem for healthcare facilities everywhere. The same precautions that you use to control infection will help safeguard you against this deadly virus. The HIV virus can ONLY pass through an exchange of body fluids. This means that normal contact with residents will not put you at risk, as long as you follow Standard Precautions when handling open wounds and fluids; touching or hugging cannot pass the disease.

TOPIC #2

Fire and Emergency Procedures

TAKE NOTE: Take this time to have your facility's safety officer or yourself review the fire and emergency procedures for your facility. Make sure the class is clear on: the location of exits, the location and operation of fire alarms and equipment, how and where to evacuate residents, and the CNA's role in the case of a fire or emergency.

To begin, SAY:

Who knows where the nearest fire alarm is? And where is the closest fire extinguisher?... For a nursing facility, a fire or other emergency can be a very hazardous situation. As you know, many residents are disabled and bedridden, and they would rely on you during any kind of emergency that required them to be moved to safety. The most important thing is to know your facility's fire and emergency procedures. This includes the placement and operation of fire alarms and extinguishing equipment, knowing what fire hazards to look for, knowing how and where to move residents, and the roles of staff in a fire emergency.

Always remember to stay calm. Immediate action is called for in an emergency and can only be executed if you are calm and confident in your emergency procedures.You should always refer to your facility's guidelines first, but here are some general things you should know about fire safety.

There are four simple steps to keep in mind in case of a fire. Using the word RACE, the steps are mapped out in the order that you should perform them.

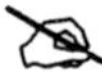

WRITE on the board:

R-A-C-E　R escue

A larm

C ontain

E xtinguish

READ the explanations for each word:

Rescue the residents who are in immediate danger (i.e., those in wheelchairs, those who are bedridden, and those with physical disabilities).

If you detect a fire, immediately sound the **Alarm.**

Contain the fire by closing all doors and windows. If you smell smoke or feel a hot door, do not open it. Also, shut off all oxygen machines. Oxygen is highly flammable.

Extinguish the fire with an extinguisher, if possible. For a grease, oil, or electrical fire, DO NOT USE WATER. Water should only be used on paper, wood, or cloth fires.

DISTRIBUTE Handout 1-3: Types of Fire Extinguishers.

After reviewing the handout, SAY:

Remember your best tools in any emergency situation are your knowledge of proper procedures and your composure. The residents are counting on you to stay calm and help them stay safe.

The above section on "Fire and Emergency Procedures" was, in part, based on the following: *The Long Term Care Nursing Assistant Training Manual* by Mary Ann Anderson, Kara W. Beaver, and Ruth E. Wheeler, Baltimore; Health Professions Press, 1991. pgs. 217-24 and *Nursing Assistants: A Basic Study Guide* by Beverly Robertson, Washington; First Class Books, Inc., 1997. pgs. 96-8.

TOPIC #3

Stopping Resident Falls

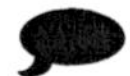

To begin, SAY:

Residents fall for various reasons. The two main groupings are: falls that happen due to a resident's mental, physical or medical condition, and falls due to a hazardous environment. You are in closer contact with the residents than most other staff members, so you will often be the first to see changes in a resident's balance or strength. Also, you can help ensure that a resident's environment is free from hazards. Remember that more than 70% of falls happen in a resident's room and bathroom, so be especially aware of these places.

DISTRIBUTE Handout 1-4: Why Do Residents Fall?

After looking over the handout, have each class member discuss a resident that they've had, who was at a significant risk of falling for any of the reasons listed in the handout. What solutions can they come up with to help the resident?

Then SAY:

As you've seen in your job as a CNA, an older person's condition can change overnight. A sudden impairment of balance, hearing, or vision, even a mild stroke can put the resident at a higher risk of falling. Also, medications can have side effects like weakness, dizziness, drowsiness, and confusion, which may lead to a greater risk of falls.

You and your co-workers need to communicate about changes in a resident so everyone is aware of that resident's level of functioning. Report changes in medication or physical condition to each other at shift changes, so that all CNAs are properly informed. Let's look at the resident's environment now.

DISTRIBUTE Handout 1-5: Environmental Risks.

Review the handout and discuss each item listed.

Then SAY:

As we've discussed, 70 percent of falls happen in the resident's room and bathroom, so keep a watchful eye on these areas. Special attention to lighting, furniture placement, and the floor and carpet conditions will also help reduce the risk of falls.

Many resident falls occur as a result of the resident attempting to toilet her or himself. Having a scheduled toileting plan in place for at-risk residents will help in reducing the number of falls.

Looking to the floor can be your best prevention against falls. When an older person sees an item on the floor, they often want to try to pick it up. As their balance is often not the best, they will probably fall. The frayed edge of a rug, a power cord, or slippery wood and linoleum floors can all be potential hazards found on the floor.

Wheelchairs are a major culprit in resident falls. The rule is that any wheelchair not being used should be locked. A stubborn resident, reluctant to ask for help, may often reach for a wheelchair. While trying to be seated, the unlocked chair can roll away, leaving the resident on the floor. A wheelchair is often used for support and if it is unlocked, the resident will often fall.

A less obvious falling hazard is badly fitting clothes and shoes. A gown or robe that is too long can cause a resident to trip. Sleeves that are too big or long can catch on things. Worn out shoes with uneven soles or squeaky new shoes with slick soles can also lead to serious falls.

When you understand the physical, medical, and environmental risks of falls, you can help residents avoid them. The more safe an environment you can offer, the lower the possibility of a fall. For residents who have fallen, you should offer encouragement in helping them regain their physical independence.

A resident who has recently fallen may see it as a foreboding sign. They may fear further injuries or feel isolated and depressed due to their newly restricted physical state. Show them you have confidence in their ability to recover. A little encouragement can make all the difference in their recovery.

A fall can be a frightening event with major consequences for a resident. By being aware of their personal condition, as well as the conditions of their surroundings, you can help keep your residents safe from falls. After a fall, look around to see why it happened and think of ways you could prevent this from occurring again.

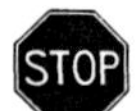

TAKE A BREAK.

TOPIC #2

Safe Body Mechanics and Transfers

For Instructor Only

Working in a nursing facility can take a heavy toll on one's physical health, not to mention one's mental and emotional health. Many of a CNA's duties require hard physical labor, like transferring residents and moving equipment. This kind of work puts CNAs at a high risk for back injuries. Researchers say that CNAs may be at a higher risk than even construction workers!

Back injuries can be extremely painful and hard to recover from, but luckily they are easy to prevent with a little work. Keeping your body in shape, understanding good body mechanics, and using proper lifting techniques can keep the back strong and injury-free.

Basic body mechanics are the key to reducing injury during resident transfers. When muscles are pushed to do things they are not equipped for, back and neck injuries result. Knowing how to use your body and the equipment, as well as being able to ask for a little help, will lead to successful transfers.

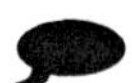

To begin, SAY:

Many people believe that back injuries are the result of a single incident; "My back just gave out," or "I hurt myself moving a resident today." This is usually not true. Researchers say that generally multiple factors lead to back injuries — factors that can be prevented.

You don't have to be a champion weightlifter to be able to lift heavy weights with minimal injury. You just need to develop a little communication between your brain and body to help prevent problems. It is far easier to prevent a back injury than to fix one, and it's also less painful.

Most of the time, people in poor physical condition will get back injuries. Bad posture, unhealthy habits, and generally being "out of shape" can place you at a greater risk of injury. You don't have to do long, daily work-outs, but maintaining normal strength and flexibility will go a long way in keeping you free from injury.

A few easy exercises, done in spare moments during your day, can help tone and condition the muscle groups you will need for lifting and transferring. They can help stretch muscle groups in your back, abdomen, leg, and arms. The few moments you take to keep these muscles in shape will prevent much longer periods of pain in the future.

So what are the top causes of back injury?

DISTRIBUTE Handout 1-6: Back Injury: The Top Causes.

Review the handout, then try the following exercise.

A Hot Idea

For a Class Exercise

Preparation before class will be required. Take various empty containers, fill them with wadded newspaper, and tape them shut. Label each one in big writing: 25 lbs., 50 lbs., 100 lbs., 200 lbs., 300 lbs., the larger the box, the higher the imaginary weight. Put the boxes around the room, place them in closets, on shelves, under beds, and on the floor.

Now, tell a class member to do exactly as you instruct them. Tell them to pick up certain boxes in certain places. Have them describe each step of their move to the class as they perform it. You and the group should coach or correct them when necessary. Monitor their body mechanics and technique. Make sure they are aware of which objects would require assistive devices to be lifted.

Then SAY:

Transferring actual people is a lot different than pretending to move heavy boxes. Moving a resident who is disabled can be one of the hardest parts of your job. If you practice good technique, good planning, and are physically prepared, you can minimize the risk of injury for you and your resident.

Ask the class what the first step of a safe transfer should be? Let them offer ideas. The right answer is to ***Greet the Resident.*** *When someone comes up with this answer, or if they fail to, write it on the board.*

DISTRIBUTE Handout 1-7: Five Steps to a Safe Transfer.

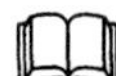

READ the five steps in the handout aloud.

Review each step with the class. When you discuss Step 2, on the importance of planning, begin a discussion of transfer equipment.

DISTRIBUTE Handout 1-8: Know Your Transfer Equipment.

Explain how to use each item on the list: If possible, have the equipment on hand and demonstrate how to use it.

Then SAY:

Most CNAs' back injuries are caused by twisting and bending at the same time. This usually happens while transferring a resident from bed to chair or from chair to bed. Let me remind you about the pivot transfer, which can save you from pain and possible injury.

DISTRIBUTE Handout 1-9: The Pivot Transfer.

Ask for two volunteers to demonstrate the pivot transfer as you read each step out loud.

Next SAY:

The pivot transfer is only to be used when a resident can cooperate with you, and when you know you can do it alone (without a co-worker). So what about residents who need more assistance? What can we do with them?

Have two class members come up at a time and role-play a resident and a CNA. Use a wheelchair, a bed, a gurney, a regular chair, etc... and have them attempt different transfers. The catch is each "resident" will have a certain medical condition or disability that makes the transfer tricky. For instance, the resident's condition might include Alzheimer's, deafness or blindness, aggression, or a weakness in one of their sides. After each pair is done, ask the class:

- *Did the CNA plan the move thoroughly?*
- *Did the CNA practice good body mechanics?*
- *Did the CNA communicate well with their resident?*
- *Did the CNA ask for help or use equipment, if necessary?*
- *What other techniques or equipment could the CNA have used?*

Then ask each "resident" these questions:

- *Did you feel secure or fearful during the transfer?*
- *Did you feel encouraged to help out?*
- *Was your final position comfortable?*

To continue, SAY:

A transfer is never over until the resident is comfortable and safe in their destination. They should be well balanced on their chair or placed squarely on their bed. A successful transfer is complete once the resident is securely positioned in their new location and their clothes have been adjusted or smoothed out, if necessary.

To conclude, DISTRIBUTE Handout 1-10: QUIZ for Module 1.

Answers to the Module 1 Quiz:

1. *False*
2. *True*
3. *True*
4. *False*
5. *False*
6. *True*
7. *False*
8. *False*
9. *False*
10. *True*

MODULE 2

Teamwork and Cooperation

Objectives of this Module

CNAs will:

- Achieve a greater understanding of the concept of teamwork and how an effective team functions
- See their central role in good caregiving
- Explore the benefits and responsibilities of teamwork, especially as it relates to staff from other departments
- Learn about the other departments' functions and responsibilities

Introduction

For Instructor Only

It seems that all types of businesses — from tiny mom and pop grocery stores to giant corporate chains — are reorganizing so that teams, instead of individuals, are responsible for meeting the company's goals. Hospitals, nursing homes, and other healthcare providers are joining in, too.

Nursing facilities need to commit to team-building, especially when it comes to the daily care of the resident and the smooth interaction of the various staff members. CNAs *know the residents as individuals and should be a part of every caregiving decision in some way. The entire facility touches the lives of residents daily through these* CNAs, *which is why they are such an integral part of good caregiving.*

TAKE NOTE: *For this module you will need participation from representatives ofdifferent departments. The idea is to form a panel from as many of the departments in your facility as possible to make a simple presentation to your class and engage them in discussion (see* Topic #4: *"The Interdisciplinary Team"). This will require some preparation beforehand; you may find* Handout 2-7: *"Tips for Panelists" helpful in this effort.*

TOPIC #1

What is Teamwork?

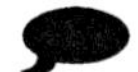

To begin, SAY:

Teamwork is important for a number of reasons. Many jobs are too large or complex for one person. Teams are a better way to solve problems because they use a wider range of people's experience, skills, and knowledge. Plus, being on a team just makes the work more fun!

In addition to performing the various tasks of being a CNA, being a cooperative and committed member of many different teams is an important part of your job, perhaps the most important part. Primarily, there is probably one partner that you work with most of the time. The rest of your team includes the charge nurse, the activities coordinator, and the other caregivers on your floor. You might be part of the team whose job it is to bathe residents, or help them at mealtime. Remember that you are also a member of an even larger team that includes your facility's administrator, director of nurses, staff development coordinator, medical director, dietary and housekeeping staff.

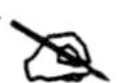

WRITE <u>What is a Team?</u> on the board.

As the group starts to come up with their definition, offer questions that will guide them to a definition similar to the following:

"A team is a group of people with many different skills, talents, and experiences, working toward a shared goal."

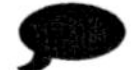

To continue, SAY:

Imagine a football team made up of eleven wide receivers or a basketball team of five centers. Little would be accomplished, because all the players share one specific skill set, and the team would lose the benefits of other players in their respective positions. On a good team, players combine their individual talents and skills for the good of everyone. Together, individual strengths and weaknesses are balanced and the whole is strengthened.

WRITE on the board:

T ogether

E veryone

A chieves

M ore

Then SAY:

As those who have played on athletic teams know, teamwork highlights the fact that others are depending on us. It also gives us colleagues that we can depend on. Teams don't just magically appear. They are slowly created — out of shared expectations of each other, common aims, and trust.

WRITE on the board:

Respect

Communication

Participation

Humor

To continue, SAY:

On a team, each member must be granted equal **respect** because everyone on the team is needed to reach the goal. This does not necessarily mean that each person's opinion is always valued the same. Some people have expertise in certain areas that other people don't have. Your expertise is in the individualized daily care of the resident.

Good **communication** begins with good listening. Listening well shows respect for the speaker and encourages him or her to continue. A good communicator asks questions to show that she is listening, as well as expressing herself clearly in her responses. Good communication skills are imperative for any individual to be an active, productive member of a team.

You are the person directly responsible for the daily care and quality of life of the resident. You know the most about them personally, which is valuable information for the rest of your team. So, **participate!** You are the expert in the daily care of the residents and should feel confident voicing your thoughts and observations.

Humor and laughter are helpful for the work of most any team, particularly in a stressful environment. Laughter is positive energy, helping you enjoy the hard work you do. It says, "We're in this together" and lifts everyone's spirits. Laughter is a reminder that, though the work you do is very serious, you don't always have to take yourself too seriously.

DISTRIBUTE Handout 2-1: The Center of the Team.

Review the handout, then SAY:

A strong team can reach their goal and work smoothly as a unit by coordinating members' different skills and responsibilities. As always, the resident's well-being is the common goal for any nursing home team.

As a CNA, you are part of the clinical, or caregiving, team, along with RNs, LPNs, various therapists, and your facility's Medical Director. But you are also part of a larger team comprised of the entire nursing facility. Your teammates — administrators, housekeeping, maintenance, medical records, billing, dietary, social services, and the residents' families — all have their own roles to play in the resident's care.

A Hot Idea

For a Class Exercise

Create small groups of four or five CNAs. Ask them to think about what is important to know in order to work most effectively with each of the departments shown on Handout 2-1. Have them write down specific questions that they would like asked of these various departments. Have one person make a list of all the questions, with a separate piece of paper for each department. Have your class use these lists during the classroom discussion with your panel of representatives later in this module (see "The Interdisciplinary Team").

TOPIC #2

Team Functions

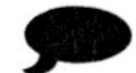

To begin, SAY:

Now, knowing who your various team members are, you should be able to understand the functions of any team. A team has five major functions, and knowing what they are and how they relate to each other is essential to the success of your team as a whole.

DISTRIBUTE Handout 2-2: The Five Functions of a Team.

Look over the handout and discuss each of the five functions as it applies to the caregiving team.

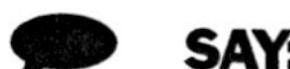

SAY:

A well-functioning team operates around three principles: trust, balance, and professionalism.

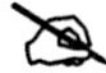

WRITE on board:

Trust

Balance

Professionalism

To continue, SAY:

Trust — Every member of a team is capable of doing their job well, if they are working in an environment where everyone is working towards a common goal and no one is trying to succeed at another team member's expense. Trust in your fellow team members will foster a healthy working environment.

Balance — On a team, the strengths and weaknesses of each member must balance out one another to make the entire group stronger.

Professionalism — Professionalism is the pride we take in our work. It includes not only how we relate to residents and their families, but also how we treat our fellow staff members.

TOPIC #3

Setting Team Goals

To begin, SAY:

A goal is an objective that your team wants to reach. On a sports team, the goal is clear: to win the game. In the nursing home, goals are more complicated. The primary goal, of course, is to ensure the resident's safety and quality of care, but there are many other important goals that need to be achieved as well.

There are two parts to any goal:

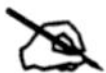

WRITE on the board:

1. Deciding on a particular objective.

2. Getting the team united to work toward that objective.

SAY:

Goals need to be carefully thought out. The first step is thinking about what you want to accomplish, and the key is to keep it attainable and realistic. When necessary, a team should not be afraid to modify or change its goal over time if its objective is not attainable.

When formulating a goal, think of the word SMART.

DISTRIBUTE Handout 2-3: Think SMART.

READ the handout to the class:

Specific — Be as clear and specific as you can about the goal.

Measurable — There should be a way to tell whether or not you have reached the goal.

Attainable — Set high goals but not too high; make sure it is a goal you can reach.

Realistic — The goal should take into account your resources, and the strengths and weaknesses of the team.

Timely — The goal should be formed so that it can be accomplished within several months, and in no longer than a year.

To continue, SAY:

Here is an example of a good goal versus a bad goal. What are the differences between the first and the second?

1. The team will make residents happier.
2. The team will improve resident satisfaction, based on scores from a survey of residents.

The first goal is too vague and not easily measurable. The second states a specific way to measure if the goal is working.

Announce a 15-minute break and remind the group that after the break members from the other departments will be visiting.

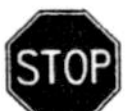

TAKE A BREAK.

TOPIC #4

The Interdisciplinary Team

Take Note: Assemble your panel of department representatives.

Introduce each of the panelists and thank them for being part of the program. Remind everyone that after the presentations there will be a question and discussion period.

To begin, SAY:

Your facility depends on you in your role as a CNA. We depend on your skills, knowledge, compassion, and personal integrity. You are the one directly responsible for the daily care and quality of life of the resident. You are the person in the facility who knows each resident's needs, hopes, fears, and abilities. You can note subtle changes in mood, behavior, appetite, and general condition that may signal the need for intervention by other members of your team. You are central to the caregiving team. The rest of your team can benefit from what you have to say.

To successfully work on a team, you need to know the other members — who they are, what their role is, and how you can work with them to help the residents. So I've asked your teammates to come in today to tell us about themselves and how they can help you in your role as a CNA.

First, I'd like you to meet ____________________ .

When all of the panelists have finished their presentations, refer the class to their lists of questions which they developed as part of "A Hot Idea" earlier in this module. Have each group ask one question that was not addressed in the presentations until they run out of questions or time.

End the unit with a group exercise. Choose from either of the exercises below, or do both. Try to make everyone participate, even if they may think it's silly or embarrassing at first. Laughter is allowed, actually, recommended.

TAKE NOTE: For these group exercises to be most effective, the panelists should be strongly encouraged to participate.

1. SALT AND PEPPER

Divide the class into pairs. Have each group come up with a compound word (such as sunshine or beanbag) or pair of related words (salt and pepper, peanut butter and jelly). They should assign one part of the word(s) to one person and the other word(s) to the other person (e.g., one is "salt" and the other is "pepper"). Now have the pairs split up and go to separate sides of the room, at least 20 feet apart. Partners should not stand directly across from one another. Now, everyone should close their eyes and start calling out their assigned word. The pairs will find each other by shouting out their word fragments, until they are together again. This is a fun way to create a sense of partnership and teamwork, while using communication skills.

2. FEED ME

Have the group split into two halves and tell participants that they should act as if their arms were in a splint (i.e., no one can bend their elbows). Have both groups sit in a circle and place a large platter of food (fruit, donuts, candy) in the middle of each circle. Now, everyone has to feed another person; everyone must have something to eat and all must be satisfied with their snack at the end. As they try to help each other fulfill this basic need — eating — they will be practicing interdependence, which involves good communication and teamwork.

A Hot Idea

For a Class Exercise

Distribute Handout 2-4: Mrs. Jones and Handout 2-5: A Sample Care Plan.

Have the class carefully look over Handout 2-4 and spend the following week asking staff from other departments questions and conferring with each other to determine how Mrs. Jones should be cared for. Have the participants devise an interdisciplinary care plan for Mrs. Jones, and bring it to the next class for feedback and discussion. If you wish, have your class use Handout 2-5 to write up their care plan.

If the above scenario isn't possible, try the following instead. Using the same two handouts, bring several facility representatives to the class who would normally be involved in devising care plans. Have volunteers from the class present Mrs. Jones to the representatives. Together, using Handout 2-5, devise a care plan for Mrs. Jones.

To conclude, DISTRIBUTE Handout 2-6: QUIZ for Module 2.

Answers to the Module 2 Quiz:

1. *False*
2. *True*
3. *False*
4. *True*
5. *True*
6. *True*
7. *False*
8. *True*
9. *False*
10. *True*

MODULE 3

Aging and Illness

Objectives of this Module

CNAs will:

- Understand the physical and functional changes that accompany nomal aging, and learn to distinguish these from the symptoms of disease
- Understand three diseases commonly found in older people and learn measures to address problems associated with them

Introduction

For Instructor Only

As you know, your nursing assistants care for people who were once active and independent and are now coping with restricted mobility and dependence. To be good and effective caregivers, your CNAs need compassion, patience, and understanding. But they also need, as the title of this module indicates, to understand the difference between normal aging and disease.

TOPIC #1

What is Normal Aging?

To begin, SAY:

For the older adult, it is often hard to accept that activities which were once easy are now difficult or even impossible. Nursing home residents are often coping with physical changes like weight loss, thinning hair, changing sleep patterns, stooped posture, and fatigue. At the same time, they are coping with how they feel about these changes, as well as with their emotions about their living situation as a resident in a nursing home.

But not all the difficulties that older adults face are unavoidable. Some physical, functional, and even psychological and emotional difficulties are the result of various diseases to which the elderly are especially prone.

It is important to be able to tell the difference between normal aging and symptoms of disease. Unlike the signs of normal aging, disease symptoms will often respond to treatment, and they can become worse or even life-threatening if ignored. As a nursing assistant, it is not your duty to diagnose illness. It is also not your duty to make the assumption that someone is healthy and "just old." It is, however, your responsibility to observe for signs and symptoms of illness, and report them.

First, let's look at the typical changes of aging.

DISTRIBUTE Handout 3-1: The Physical Changes of Aging

After reviewing the handout, SAY:

The attitude that certain pain and problems naturally go along with aging is a dangerous one. Some of the normal aging signs can also be disease symptoms. The physical changes of aging can mask the symptoms of disease. Use your awareness and observation skills, and ask more questions when necessary. For example, if a resident complains of pain, ask them:

WRITE on the board:

- What kind of pain is it?
- Where exactly does it hurt?
- How much does it hurt on a scale of 1-10?
- How long have you felt this way?
- Does this happen at a certain time of day?

To continue, SAY:

Think about this example. A resident complains of headaches and weakness in one arm. His speech seems confused and he has started snapping at the CNAs. All of these symptoms could be passed off as a grouchy old man, but they could also be signs of a transient ischemic attack or TIA. A TIA is a kind of mini-stroke that often precedes a real stroke. Beware of shrugging off changes in a resident that could also be disease symptoms.

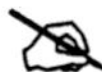

WRITE on the board:

- Fatigue
- Weight loss
- Change in sleep patterns

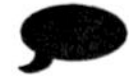

To continue, SAY:

If you saw that a resident was experiencing these three things, would you shrug it off as the effects of aging? Many caregivers would, which is why depression is often left undiagnosed in nursing homes. We'll discuss depression more in depth later in module seven.

If a possible disease symptom is not treated in a timely manner, it can spiral quickly into serious illness. Look at these four things and let's look at how they are related to one another:

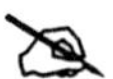

WRITE on the board:

- Incontinence
- Reduced fluid intake
- Constipation
- Sickness

Next SAY:

Repeated incontinence is always a symptom of disease. An embarrassed resident may not know this and try to reduce accidents by drinking less fluid. As fluids are necessary for proper bowel movements, the resident may become constipated. The constipation could then lead to further sickness. Again, the key is to be alert and observant. Know which symptoms might signal a disease. When in doubt, report your observations and concerns.

In addition to the many physical changes the elderly experience, it is important to note the functional changes they go through as well:

WRITE on the board:

Functional changes:

- Bowel and bladder control
- Recreation
- Mobility
- Sensory perception

To continue, SAY:

Looking at the big picture, the elderly also experience other important changes — namely, environmental changes. Living in a nursing home carries a whole new set of situations and conditions with it, such as:

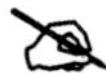

WRITE on the board:

- Unfamiliar environment
- Poor sensory environment
- Excessive stimulation
- Different communication styles
- Excessive clutter
- Inadequate orientation

SAY:

Knowledge of the difference between aging and disease can help you save your residents unnecessary pain. Understanding and compassion are equally as important; these people were once active and independent, and may have trouble accepting their new limitations.

Let's now have a look at three diseases that sometimes get mis-diagnosed as simply "being old." First, we're going to look at a disease that affects approximately one-fifth of all people over 65 — namely diabetes.

TAKE NOTE: *You might want to invite your facility's medical director to review the symptoms and treatments available for diabetes, osteoarthritis, stroke, and any other illnesses prevalent in your facility.*

TOPIC #2

Diabetes

To begin, SAY:

Diabetes is sometimes called "high blood sugar." The body needs sugar for energy, but too much sugar in the blood is damaging to the body.

Sugar is carried in the bloodstream to all the cells of the body. In order for the cells to receive and use the sugar, they must first be "unlocked" by a chemical called insulin. If the body doesn't produce enough insulin, then the sugar cannot enter the cells and remains in the blood. This high level of sugar in the blood is what we call diabetes. There are two types of diabetes.

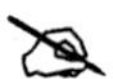

WRITE on the board:

Type I — usually begins when young

Type II — usually begins at middle age

SAY:

Type I diabetes is the result of a genetic condition that prevents the body from making insulin at all. People with Type I diabetes are usually diagnosed when they are children or teenagers. People with Type I diabetes must regularly inject insulin into their bloodstream in order to make up for their bodies' inability to produce it naturally.

Type II diabetes usually shows up in a person's middle-aged years or later. As Type II diabetics age, their bodies are less able to either produce insulin or effectively use the insulin they produce. This is the more common form of diabetes in extended care facilities. Type II diabetes is treated through diet and exercise, and sometimes medication.

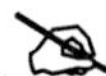

WRITE on the board:

Complications of Diabetes:

- Blindness
- Nerve damage
- Increased risk of infection
- Kidney failure
- Dental problems
- Stroke
- Heart disease
- Decreased circulation/Foot problems

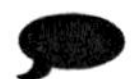

Then SAY:

Diabetes is a serious, chronic illness. In other words, it is an ongoing illness that can be treated but not cured. If not treated properly, diabetes can cause blindness, nerve damage, increased risk of infection, kidney failure, dental problems, stroke, and heart disease.

There are some warning signs you should watch for in your diabetic residents that will require immediate attention or medical assistance.

DISTRIBUTE Handout 3-2: Diabetic Warning Signs.

After discussing the handout, SAY:

So what can you do to help your diabetic residents? There are four key things.

WRITE on the board:

1. Educate yourself.

2. Educate your resident.

3. Work closely with other staff.

4. Guard against dehydration.

Then SAY:

Educate yourself.

Understanding diabetes can help you to care for your diabetic residents. Knowing the warning signs of high and low blood sugar and understanding the reasons behind the resident's dietary plan will make you a better caregiver.

Educate your resident.

As you learn about diabetes, share what you learn with the resident. Try to help the resident participate in the treatment, not just go along with it. Let the diabetic resident know you want to help him keep his blood sugar at safe levels.

Work closely with other staff.

Report any warning signs to the nurse in charge. Document food and fluid intake. Communicate information to your colleagues on the next shift. It takes a team to care for the diabetic resident effectively.

Guard against dehydration.

Dehydration is a common problem in residents of an extended care facility, but it is especially dangerous for the diabetic resident. Know the warning signs of dehydration. Encourage diabetic residents to drink plenty of sugar-free fluids throughout the day.

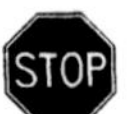

TAKE A BREAK.

TOPIC #3

Arthritis

To begin, SAY:

Let's look at another disease that commonly affects the elderly: arthritis. There are two kinds of arthritis: osteoarthritis and rheumatoid. And the one that most often afflicts the elderly is osteoarthritis.

Osteoarthritis is a disease of aging. It is the gradual deterioration of cartilage, which serves as the shock absorber in a joint. In older people this cartilage wears down, causing bone to begin scraping against bone. Needless to say, this can be very painful. Normally, joints repair themselves as they degenerate. But with osteoarthritis, the repairing doesn't keep up with the degeneration.

Usually, osteoarthritis is found in only one or two specific joints, not throughout the body. Osteoarthritis can affect the neck, knees, hips, or spine. Most frequently it affects the fingers, causing pain, stiffness, and frustration that can keep residents from enjoying activities.

So, what are the causes and symptoms of osteoarthritis?

DISTRIBUTE Handout 3-3: Osteoarthritis.

After discussing the handout, SAY:

You can help residents with osteoarthritis in many ways, including:

This may be a good time to educate your class on the proper application of braces and the proper technique for applicable ROM exercises.

WRITE on the board:

- Apply braces
- Assist with range of motion (ROM) exercises
- Encourage ambulation
- Encourage frequent rest
- Provide emotional support

SAY:

While most arthritis in long-term care facilities is osteoarthritis, you may also have to care for residents with rheumatoid arthritis. Rheumatoid arthritis affects all the joints of the body. It also impacts the tissue surrounding those joints. Unlike osteoarthritis, which has distinct causes, rheumatoid arthritis has no known cause. It is known that physical and emotional stress can bring on attacks of rheumatoid arthritis after a person has been diagnosed.

Symptoms of rheumatoid arthritis include:

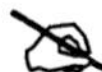 **WRITE on the board:**

- Fever
- General feeling of illness
- Weight loss
- Morning stiffness

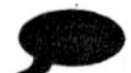 **To continue, SAY:**

As with osteoarthritis, there are ways you can help residents with rheumatoid arthritis:

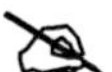 **WRITE on the board:**

- Emotional support
- Skin care to affected areas and joints
- Properly position body
- Assistive devices
- Promote independent movement

 **SAY:**

Arthritis pain can be eased by medications and assistive devices can be used for some affected areas, but the best treatment is surgery. Many of you have dealt with residents who have undergone hip surgery. Here are some specifics on how you can help them after surgery.

 **DISTRIBUTE Handout 3-4: Hip Surgery Precautions.**

Take Note: This would be a good time to demonstrate the use of an abductor wedge. If you can, also show the class a prosthetic device, such as a metal, plastic, or ceramic hip replacement piece, and how it works.

To continue, SAY:

All elderly bodies are delicate, but those who have had hip replacement need extra special care. When someone has a hip replacement, their joint is replaced with metal and plastic pieces that slide easily over one another. Your main concern for these residents should be when moving them. Never, never, never move their hip past 90 degrees; this is the cardinal rule. Make sure the hip is supported while you move them and keep their back straight as they rise.

While the resident is in bed, make sure you change their position often. This will offer relief to their muscles and bones, as well as helping prevent pressure ulcers. Keep their hip aligned with an abductor wedge while they're resting, but be sure to take it off when you move them.

TOPIC #4

Stroke

 **To begin, SAY:**

A stroke, or "brain attack," occurs when blood circulation to the brain fails. This is usually the result of a blockage, but it can also be caused by bleeding. Brain cells can die from decreased blood flow and the resulting lack of oxygen. While people of any age can suffer a stroke, the elderly — particularly those with a history of heart disease, high blood pressure, or diabetes — are at greater risk. Strokes are also more frequently fatal in older people.

There are four causes of strokes:

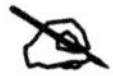 **WRITE on the board:**

1. Blockage

2. Thrombus

3. Embolus

4. Rupture

 **To continue, SAY:**

Blockage is when blood vessels get blocked and no blood gets to the brain. Thrombus is a blood clot in the brain. Embolus is a blood clot carried to the brain through the circulatory system. Rupture is bleeding in the brain.

Strokes fall under two categories: hemiplegia and hemiparesis. Hemiplegia, which mean paralysis on one side of the body, usually the opposite side of the body from the side of the brain the stroke occurred on. Hemiparesis is the other type, where movement is possible, but there is a loss of sensation in the affected side. The body sends clues or "warning signs" to the brain that it is not getting enough oxygen.

Have the class identify any residents under their care who have experienced hemiplegia or hemiparesis.

DISTRIBUTE Handout 3-5: Possible Signs of Stroke.

READ the handout out loud.

Then SAY:

Other danger signs that may occur include double vision, drowsiness, and nausea or vomiting. Sometimes the warning signs may last only a few moments and then disappear. These brief episodes, known as TIAs (transient ischemic attacks), are sometimes called "mini-strokes." Because they clear up, many people ignore them. Don't. Often they are like the mild tremors that warn of a coming earthquake. You may be saving the resident's life.

There are three stages a stroke victim goes through. They are:

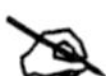

WRITE on the board:

1. Flaccid

2. Spastic

3. Recovery

Then SAY:

When stroke victims are flaccid, the affected side is limp and weak. When they are spastic, the affected side develops tense muscles and spasms. And finally, under recovery, the victim's affected side regains normal use.

So, how can you help in the treatment and recovery of stroke victims?

DISTRIBUTE Handout 3-6: Care for Stroke Patients.

READ the handout out loud.

Then SAY:

As nursing assistants, you care for people who were once active and independent, and are now coping with restricted mobility and dependence. You need compassion, patience, and understanding.

By being a careful observer of the changing condition of the residents in your care, you can often tell the difference between the normal troubles that older people experience, and the needless pain and suffering that are caused by illnesses that can be treated.

A portion of the above section on strokes was based on *Nursing Assistants: A Basic Study Guide*. 1997. First Class Books, Inc., p. 117.

A Hot Idea

For a Class Exercise

With Handout 3-1 in mind, you will now conduct nursing assistant "rounds." Make sure everyone has a pen and a notebook. Explain to the group that you are all going to leave the classroom and walk through the facility, noting the various changes that have occurred to particular residents that you have selected, as a result of the aging process.

Ask the nursing assistants to look at each of these residents and to note the physical, functional, and environmental changes associated with aging. Ask them also to note any specific disease symptoms that are present. Ask if there are any ongoing treatments to be aware of. What are they? Are there any symptoms of potential disease that should be monitored?

After the "rounds," compare notes as a group, and conduct a discussion of each resident. Use the following questions:

- Describe what you believe to be the major changes the resident has experienced over the past decade of their life.
- What specific changes do you think the resident is having the most difficult time adjusting to?
- Are there visible symptoms of disease? What are they?
- Is the resident receiving treatment for the disease?
- How would you care for this person to either prevent disease, or to keep their disease from worsening?

To conclude, DISTRIBUTE Handout 3-7: QUIZ for Module 3.

Answers to the Module 3 Quiz:

1. True

2. True

3. False

4. True

5. False

6. False

7. True

8. True

9. False

10. True

MODULE 4

Communication is Key

Objectives of this Module

CNAs will:

- Learn specific tactics for improving communication
- Discover the importance of clear communication in the facility
- Learn to identify possible impediments to open, productive communication

Introduction

For Instructor Only

CNAs deal with all types of people daily, each with their own set of needs and goals. Communication, under these circumstances, is anything but easy. In their profession as caregivers, even the best CNAs, who are great communicators and have wonderful people skills, sometimes find communication hard.

Everyone is stressed out — from the CNA to the resident to the nurse to the administrator to the family. Stress often causes people to not listen fully to each other, which can in turn lead to serious conflict. And in times of conflict, communication becomes crucial.

Good communication is a skill, and like so many other things in a CNA's round of responsibilities, can be improved with practice. This module will explore ways to listen fully and evaluate what others have to say. It will offer specific tips on clear, honest ways to express oneself. It will also discuss certain barriers to good communication and how to overcome them.

TOPIC #1

Communication Skills

 **To begin, SAY:**

Communication isn't a problem when your life and job are running smoothly. But really, how often is this the case? In the stressful world of the nursing facility, communication can sometimes be strained. We sometimes don't have the time or patience to listen fully or to clearly express our thoughts. Or we may find ourselves in conflict with a resident, family, or fellow staff member.

There are specific things you can learn to improve your communication skills, just as you learned how to transfer a resident, or how to perform your ADLs. With a few simple skills and a little practice, you will be able to better communicate, especially in those difficult situations.

"Active listening" is a key communication skill. If you think of responses before someone is done speaking, or think about what you're going to eat for lunch that day instead of what is being said, you are not being an active listener. Try to force yourself to listen to someone fully when they are speaking. First focus on what they are saying, then decide how you will answer them.

The key to successful active listening is staying calm, even when you feel stressed out or when someone is verbally attacking you. Try to figure out how the other person is feeling, what they are upset about. Try to see what the real problem behind the complaint or issue at hand might be.

When you have fully examined the situation, decide how you will respond. An angry reaction will just make the situation worse. Maybe the person just wants someone to listen to them. Try to keep some of these active listening tips in mind next time you're having trouble communicating with someone.

DISTRIBUTE Handout 4-1: Test Your Communication Skills.

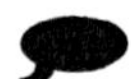

Then SAY:

Let's try taking an honest look at how we communicate. What do we do well? How can we improve our communicating style?

Start a class discussion by reading each of the statements on the handout out loud. Which statements does the group agree with? Which do they disagree with? Which seem like especially hard things to do? Why are some of the things on the handout so difficult to do? How can the particular skills listed on the handout help them communicate better?

A Hot Idea

For a Class Exercise

And now for something a little different...

Play the classic telephone game to show the importance of clear communication. The group sits in a circle. One person whispers a word or phrase into the ear of the person to his/her right, who tries to whisper what he/she heard to the next person, and so on until it has gone all the way around the circle. The last person says what he/she heard, which is often quite different from the original phrase!

TOPIC #2

Active Listening Skills

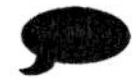 **To begin, SAY:**

In becoming better communicators, there are a few techniques you should know. These will help you be a better listener with family members, co-workers, and your residents, maybe even your own family and friends! These three aids will help you become a better listener.

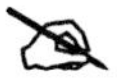 **WRITE on the board:**

3 Communication Aids:

1. Ask open questions

2. Invite

3. Encourage

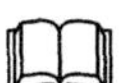 **READ to the class:**

1. Ask open questions. Ask questions that require more than a yes or no answer.

"How do you feel about Mrs. Kenan's angry outburst yesterday?"

2. Invite. Ask, never force, a person to talk to you.

"Do you want to talk about your argument with the supervisor?"

3. Encourage. Encourage the person to tell you their concerns.

"You seem upset. I'd like to hear your problem if you want to talk."

Ask the class if anyone remembers a time they used one of these communication aids. If they can't come up with any, offer some yourself.

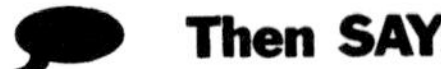

Then SAY:

These three communication aids can work wonders, especially with resident's family members. With this in mind, we should also list some of the things that can prevent good communication.

DISTRIBUTE Handout 4-2: Communication Roadblocks.

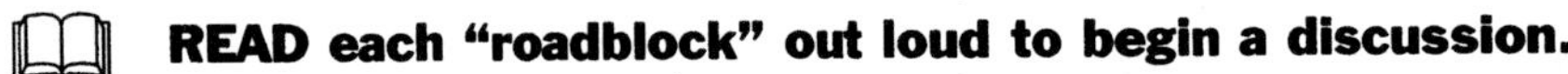

READ each "roadblock" out loud to begin a discussion.

Lead the class discussion with these questions:

- *Have you ever encountered these roadblocks?*
- *Which communication aid could have helped in these cases?*
- *Can anyone think of another communication roadblock?*
- *When you encountered one of these roadblocks, were you less willing to communicate?*

After a brief discussion, SAY:

So, we've looked at ways to initiate or improve conversation, as well as some blocks to good conversation. Remember, it isn't enough to stand still and let the person talk at you, you need to actively listen. This means showing the person you understand what they are saying — verbally and non-verbally.

Another listening skill that you practice every day in your job is following directions. Try this fun little exercise to see how good you are at following directions.

Distribute Handout 4-3: Follow The Yellow Brick Road.

TOPIC #3

Feedback

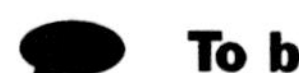

To begin, SAY:

To let a speaker know that you have understood them, there are different things you can do. First, give a summary of what they've said, and then offer personal responses or possible solutions. Giving good feedback is just one of the many things that will make you a good communicator. Here are three kinds of feedback.

DISTRIBUTE Handout 4-4: Three Types of Feedback.

READ the handout to the class.

Have two members of the class act out a discussion. Have one present a problem and the other offer one of the kinds of feedback for that problem. Try this with a few pairs in the class and discuss the effectiveness of their feedback.

To continue, SAY:

All three kinds of feedback can be helpful in different ways. Emotion-based feedback can be an excellent way to show a person you understand how they feel about a problem. This is another way to re-enforce that you are actively listening to a person. Something like, "I understand that you feel bad about your mother's sickness. It must be really hard." If the person is feeling edgy or under attack, an emotional feedback could put them at ease.

Fact-based feedback basically shows the person that you are listening and that you understand their problem. If used later in a conversation, it can also help solidify a decision that you have come to together; for example, "You'll call if you're not going to visit your mother next week, so we can warn her and keep her from having another crying episode."

When providing feedback regarding someone's concern or problem, you should always strive to move toward a solution. This is what we mean by solution-based feedback. It's a way to sum up the conversation and allow you to work together with the other person in finding a solution. After someone has told you the problem and you have offered your feedback, sum up what you think has been said. This will help clarify each person's side and make it easier to find a solution.

It's very frustrating to feel that someone is not really listening to you. If you are already upset or stressed about a problem, a poor listener will only make you feel worse. Since you know how bad being ignored or misunderstood feels, be extra careful to actively listen when people come to you with problems.

TOPIC #4

I-Messages

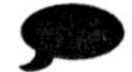

To begin, SAY:

Another good tool to use is called an "I-message." Using "I" instead of "you" shows the person you are not blaming them. When a person feels blamed or accused, they may jump on the defensive. The "I-message" is a way to say what you mean without upsetting the other person. Look at this sentence: "You are so inconsiderate! You never tell us when you're going to be late for work." What other type of communication roadblock is being used here?

DISTRIBUTE Handout 4-5: "I-Messages."

As you pass out the handout, SAY:

Using "always" or "never" is a generalization and does not help good communication. So when a person hears "you" and feels blamed, they will jump on the defensive and probably not listen to your complaint. An "I-message" would be more effective in this situation.

So, what exactly does an "I-message" look like?

An I-message starts by stating your problem, in a non-blaming way.

> "When you yell at me about your mother's missing dress..."

It continues by telling the other person how it makes you feel and why.

> "I feel hurt and accused, because we try really hard to keep track of everyone's laundry."

If you have a solution, state it now.

> "Maybe we can re-sew labels onto her clothes, because many are missing them."

If you have no solution, try one of the communication aids you learned earlier.

> "I would like us both to feel better. Can we try talking about this?"

No matter what the solution, thank them for listening to your viewpoint. This could help pave the way for good future communication between the two of you.

Remember: The key to I-messages is not blaming or judging the other person. Don't try to approach the problem when you are at the height of your anger. A highly emotional state will not help you communicate well. If you discuss your problem calmly and clearly, generally the other person will be more willing to try to find a solution.

A Hot Idea

For a Class Exercise

Try this role-play exercise.

Go back and review the communication skills you have learned up to this point. Discuss communication aids and roadblocks, active listening, feedback, and I-messages. Now get two volunteers from the class. Have one play a "family member" and have one play a "CNA". Take one of the scenarios below and have them act it out. Let the class coach them as they go along. Make sure they use as many of the skills and aids that they've learned up to this point as possible.

After this situation has been acted out, get two more volunteers. Have them play a pair of "staff members" in conflict. Again, let the rest of the class help out and make sure they are using the communication skills they have learned.

Here are a few conflict scenarios to choose from:

- A staff member arrives late for work and does not apologize.
- A family member is unable to make a scheduled visit to their relative.
- A family member is rude to a CNA because their loved one has not been bathed.
- A staff member does not help with the residents at mealtime.

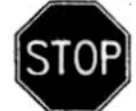

TAKE A BREAK.

TOPIC #5

Communication Challenges

For Instructor Only

The nursing facility and world we live in change more every day. With so many different kinds of people, the potential for conflict grows. The conflict is often between people's different cultural values. If we can learn to understand and accept the varying cultures and values around us, communication will become much easier.

Differences in cultural values can lead to serious communication problems in the nursing facility. Staff members will often have different ideas about their residents, how much attention to give them, how close to be with them, how much freedom they should be allowed, etc... Cultural and religious differences can be especially frustrating (as we will see in Module 6). To work in a nursing facility, staff and residents need to continue to try to understand each other's values.

It is inevitable, with so many staff members and residents that there will be conflicting religious and ethnic associations. A resident from a certain ethnic group may have prejudices or strong beliefs that clash with those of another resident or staff member. A resident and a staff member may have conflicting religious beliefs. With good communication, many of these problems can be overcome.

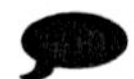

To begin, SAY:

Cultural differences can be a big problem in the nursing home. With so many values, morals, and beliefs in one place, there is bound to be conflict. Residents and staff may differ in religion, ethnic backgrounds, or personal morality. Some people carry prejudices along with these beliefs, even stereotypes about those that have other beliefs.

Good communication is key when all of these values and cultures collide. We need to understand and accept each other's values if we're going to get along.

So what makes up a culture? It's not just different clothes, music, and food. It is also a different way of interacting with the world and a different language. It is made up of a set of behaviors, attitudes, values, and beliefs that define that particular group.

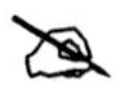

WRITE on the board:

A culture is a set of:

- behaviors
- attitudes
- values
- beliefs

DISTRIBUTE Handout 4-6: Tony and Mrs. Li.

Look over the handout and then review the definition of culture again. Ask the class if Tony and Mrs. Li are experiencing a conflict of cultures. Is Mrs. Li upset with Tony or is this her cultural response to this situation? Emphasize that many problems between people from different cultures are simply misunderstandings.

To continue, SAY:

In this story, Tony offended Mrs. Li by being so open and informal. She comes from a Japanese culture, where unknown men should not look a woman in the eye, address her by her first name, or attempt physical contact with her. Tony was unknowingly being disrespectful. In addition to being confused and insulted by his greeting, Mrs. Li is not at liberty to tell a strange man of his error.

Tony comes from a very different cultural background. As a native New Yorker with Italian heritage, he is used to being loud and informal is his natural state with people. Greeting someone formally would seem forced and unfriendly to him.

As a CNA, you need to know about your resident's different cultural backgrounds. It can help your interactions and communication with them run more smoothly. Knowing how your culture has affected you will also help you interact with people of other cultures better.

We all want to be understood and accepted for who we are. Your residents and co-workers feel the same way. Knowing about each other's cultural backgrounds will help our communication with each other. Handling these cultural differences can be a really tough job, but it is a necessary one. In your position as a CNA, you can help build a setting of cultural exchange, where everyone feels appreciated.

DISTRIBUTE Handout 4-7: Cultural Communication Tips.

Review the handout and ask the class to give examples of each communication tip listed. They should use examples from their work or personal lives. Discuss the difference between verbal communication and body language in different cultures. Ask for examples. Tell them that body language can be as powerful as verbal language, and a gesture may mean very different things in different cultures.

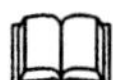

READ the following scenario to the class:

A Native American CNA works in a Catholic nursing facility. She wants to take the day off from work on Thursday, as it is one of her tribe's holy days. Her supervisor says no immediately, without hearing out her request. He tells her that her sick days are already used up and if she misses another day, for any excuse, her job will be in question. She feels that her supervisor is not listening or being sensitive to her dilemma.

Ask the class how they would react? What cultural difference is causing the conflict? How would they solve it?

DISTRIBUTE Handout 4-8: Betty and Maureen.

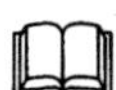

READ over the handout with the class.

Ask them to think about this scenario for a few minutes and to come up with a solution. What would be a better way for Maureen to present her problem? Have them construct an I-message for Maureen to use.

To conclude, DISTRIBUTE Handout 4-9: Quiz for Module 4.

Answers to the Module 4 Quiz:

1. *True*
2. *False*
3. *True*
4. *False*
5. *True*
6. *False*
7. *True*
8. *False*
9. *True*
10. *False*

MODULE 5

Nutrition

Objectives of this Module

CNAs will:

- Learn the basics of good nutrition and hydration for older adults
- Be alert to the warning signs of nutritional problems and the conditions of nutritional risk
- Learn factors that affect eating ability and appetite

Introduction

For Instructor Only

Dietitians and nurses are primarily responsible for resident's nutrition in a facility, but CNAs must do their part as well. If CNAs know the basics of good nutrition and hydration, as well as nutritional risk factors, they can aid the dietary and nursing staff in their job. Since CNAs work closely with the residents, they act as an important safeguard against a resident's nutritional problems.

TAKE NOTE: The participation of dietitians and nurses from your facility would be useful in this module. Ideally, they should come to address the class about nutrition, how it relates to their jobs, and the CNAs' job. If there is not a convenient time for this, ask them for some exercises or ideas on the subject that you can present to the class.

To introduce this module, SAY:

Good nutrition is important for everyone, but it is crucial for older people. Although you are not dietitians, you can aid in a resident's good eating habits by knowing the basics of good nutrition, watching for eating problems, and encouraging them to eat well. As you know, residents often need advice on healthy eating choices and the encouragement to actually eat sometimes. Other residents need physical assistance to feed themselves.

Aside from being a keen observer and advisor on residents' nutrition, you must ensure that the food and social eating environment appeal to the resident. We will look at different aspects of food, hydration, and nutrition. Also, we'll talk about nutritional problems and warning signs, and ways to help a resident keep up a healthy appetite.

TOPIC #1

Good Nutrition Basics

To begin, SAY:

Practicing good nutrition means knowing the proper amounts of these five things: fruits and vegetables, dairy, fiber, protein, and, most importantly, water. Let's start with fruits and vegetables.

WRITE Fruits and Vegetables on the board.

SAY:

This can be the most fun part of a good diet. Fruit is nature's candy; it's good for us and it tastes good. Vegetables are colorful, tasty, and provide us with many of the major vitamins we need.

WRITE 3 servings of Vegetables, 2 servings of Fruit on the board.

To continue, SAY:

At least three servings of vegetables and two of fruit are recommended per day. Did you know that the darker the vegetable is, the more nutrients it has? Keep this in mind when you monitor a resident's meals. Are they getting enough fruits and vegetables? If not, how can you change this?

Allow for class answers, then WRITE on board:

- Spinach
- Broccoli
- Mustard Greens
- Cauliflower
- Kale

SAY:

The vegetables in the cabbage family are rich in cancer-blocking chemicals. Think about what I said earlier about darker colored vegetables. Which on this list are packed with nutrients, as well as having cancer-blocking properties?

Allow class to answer, then SAY:

Fresh fruits and vegetables are preferable, but frozen and canned can be acceptable. Fruit in canned syrup is not good. Why would this be?

Allow class to answer, then SAY:

Canned syrup means extra sugar. Residents should avoid any food high in sugar. Sugar satisfies the appetite, but gives no nutritional benefit. It gives quick calories, but no vitamins or minerals. It may be quick and fulfill a resident's craving, but it can lead to malnutrition if used as a substitute for other foods.

WRITE Dairy, Calcium, and Vitamin D on the board.

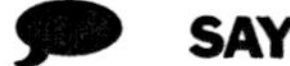

SAY:

Most adults, and especially older adults, do not get the proper amounts of calcium or vitamin D. They should have three servings a day and preferably low fat ones, like yogurt, skim milk, and hard cheese. Calcium fortified orange juice and calcium supplements are also a good way to make sure your residents get their daily amount.

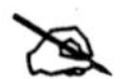

WRITE <u>Fiber</u> on the board.

Then SAY:

Fiber helps the digestive system absorb nutrients from other food, as well as having many important nutrients. Bread, rice, pasta, and cereal, made from whole grains, are great sources. Fiber can help residents in many ways:

WRITE on the board:

- <u>Protects against cancer</u>
- <u>Prevents constipation</u>
- <u>Keeps blood sugar levels normal</u>
- <u>Fights high cholesterol</u>

READ each item aloud as you write them.

WRITE <u>Protein</u> on the board.

SAY:

Our bodies use protein to build muscle and without it we become frail and weak. Elders especially need this and can get it through lean poultry and meats, fish, and dried beans. Dried beans offer both high protein and lots of fiber. Fish can also help lessen heart attack risk.

WRITE Water on the board.

ASK the class:

What happens to the body without enough water?

WRITE on the board:

- Medications can build up in kidneys, making a resident very ill
- Blood pressure falls dangerously low
- Blood clots form and block blood vessels to the heart
- Chronic constipation

READ each item aloud as you write them.

To continue, SAY:

Eight 8-ounce glasses of water a day are recommended. Non-caffeinated soda is also good, non-caffeinated because caffeine takes fluid away from the body. Alcohol, as well as caffeine, has the effect of taking away the body's hydration, or acts as a diuretic.

Now review the items on the list and have the class tell you the benefits of each basic nutritional building block.

Offer these questions to help lead a discussion of the basics of good nutrition:

- *How many servings of vegetables are recommended daily?*
- *How many servings of fruit are recommended daily?*
- *Why are vegetables in the cabbage family especially good for you?*
- *Why are fruits in canned syrup bad?*
- *Which two important nutrients are found in dairy?*
- *What are some good sources of fiber?*
- *Why is fiber so important?*
- *What does protein do for your body?*
- *How many glasses of water are recommended per day?*
- *What can happen to the body without enough water?*
- *Why are caffeinated and alcoholic beverages not acceptable forms of hydration?*

DISTRIBUTE Handout 5-1: The Pyramid of Food.

Then SAY:

You've probably seen this food pyramid hundreds of times, on cereal boxes and in books. Keep it now as a reference tool to help you think about your residents' nutrition.

If your class needs additional help understanding the information in Handout 5-1, try this exercise: Have the class break up into two groups and develop a menu for one day using the food pyramid.

TOPIC #2

Nutritional Problems in the Elderly

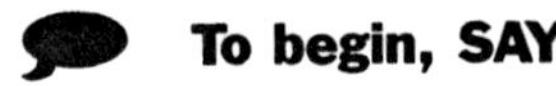

To begin, SAY:

Malnutrition is a big problem according to the U.S. Department of Health. In one survey they found that between 35 and 50 percent of residents in long term care facilities were malnourished! Some of the harmful effects of malnutrition include: weight loss or obesity, decreased ability to fight disease, and reduced strength. If a resident suffers from dementia, malnutrition can make them more confused and disoriented.

DISTRIBUTE Handout 5-2: Symptoms of Nutritional Disease.

Review handout and then SAY:

Looking at this handout, we see that nutrition can have effects on every part of a person's physical and mental health. When a problem is diagnosed as nutritional, it can usually be cured without medication, by a change in diet or by adding vitamin and mineral supplements. These symptoms can be warnings of other illnesses, but nutrition must always be kept in mind as a source of problems in older adults.

How can we determine when an older person is at nutritional risk?

DISTRIBUTE Handout 5-3: The DETERMINE List.

To continue, SAY:

The Nutritional Screening Initiative developed this tool, "Checklist to DETERMINE Nutritional Health," that lists warning signs of nutritional risk. The checklist uses each letter in the word DETERMINE to remind us of these warning signs.

The DETERMINE model highlights nine major factors that lead to nutrition problems. As with your nutritional pyramid, use the DETERMINE model as an awareness tool, rather than a precise scientific measure. It can help you become aware of problems early, so you can alert a dietician or nurse, if needed. This tool can be especially useful with new residents. Many residents' nutritional problems begin before they enter a nursing home, so they are especially at risk.

So, what is your role in helping prevent nutritional risk? You have the advantage of frequent, close contact with residents, which could make you the first to notice a problem. DETERMINE will help you notice warning signs of nutritional risk early on. Along with knowing the basics of nutrition, this model can help you keep your residents in good nutritional health.

Some of the DETERMINE factors may seem obvious, like noticing when a resident is eating poorly. Many others are less obvious, like the effects of economic hardship or reduced social contact. These non-physical factors can have as great an effect as any physical one. By listing these obvious and less obvious factors, DETERMINE helps raise our awareness of nutritional risks.

Tell your nursing supervisor if you suspect a resident is at nutritional risk. They can bring in a facility dietician or the resident's physician to make a thorough examination. If the whole staff works together, the nutrition of your residents will undoubtedly improve.

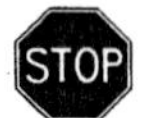

TAKE A BREAK.

The DETERMINE checklist tool comes from The Nutrition Screening Initiative's "Report of Nutrition Screening 1: Toward a Common View, Executive Summary," Washington, D.C.

TOPIC #3

Malnutrition

For those who care for the elderly, malnutrition is a major concern. Although CNAs do not prepare menus for residents, they can aid the dietary staff by having a good grasp of the basics of nutrition and malnutrition. They can also help by becoming better observers and reporters of residents' eating problems.

To begin, SAY:

What exactly does malnutrition mean? It is when a person lacks essential nutrients, water, and dietary fiber. The health of our body is directly influenced by the foods we do or do not eat, especially for the elderly. Malnutrition can lead to heart or kidney disease, and even cancer, if not treated.

You might think of hungry, poverty stricken people when you hear about malnutrition. Poverty can be a cause, but there are many other factors that can affect people, regardless of their financial situation or the amount of available food. For older people, there are some other important reasons. The first reason would be loss of appetite.

DISTRIBUTE Handout 5-4: Loss of Appetite.

Review the handout, then SAY:

As the person who deals most directly and often with the residents, you can monitor the resident's social and physical eating environments. You can observe chewing and swallowing problems, as well as pain and nausea. Work with the dietitians and nurses to ensure that their food comes at the proper temperature and time.

There is always something you can do when you recognize a resident's nutritional problem. You can report your observations to nursing or dietary staff or, perhaps, as the primary caregiver, you can try to take care of the problem yourself. How would you react to each of the problems on the list in Handout 5-4?

Allow for discussion, then DISTRIBUTE Handout 5-5: Calories.

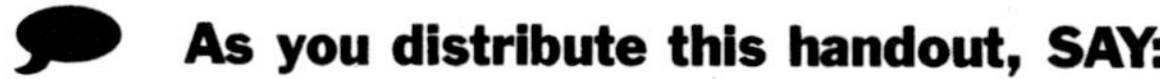

As you distribute this handout, SAY:

Malnourishment happens because people don't eat enough food or they eat food that doesn't have the proper nutrients they need. As the "Loss of Appetite" handout has shown us, older people often don't eat enough or they eat filling foods that don't have the necessary nutrients. It is important that, as a CNA, you know which foods will help residents keep up their strength and energy.

In your position, you often need to help residents make food choices. You also provide them with snacks and, at times, work with the dietary staff to determine their preferences and needs. This is an important position, in which you can directly effect the nutritional well-being of your residents.

Review the handout, then SAY:

Now that you know malnutrition isn't just about not getting enough calories, you can help your residents by offering the right amounts of healthy foods. Let's look at this handout and think about what foods we would give a resident who is not making good nutritional choices.

Separate the class into smaller groups.

Then DISTRIBUTE Handout 5-6: Mr. Parks.

Review Mr. Parks' story and ask the group these leading questions:

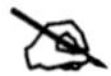 **WRITE on the board:**

- What do you think is happening to Mr. Parks?
- What other information would you need to better assess his situation?
- How would you encourage a change in his mealtime eating habits?
- What healthy snacks or desserts could you offer him?
- How could you help him regain good nutrition?

Each group should confer and report their answers. Make sure they have accounted for his history, recent illness, and medication. Stress the importance of the dietary department and communication among staff about his situation.

 **To continue, SAY:**

Before we move onto the social aspect of food, let me stress again the importance of water. Dehydration can have extremely harmful effects on a weak resident. Make sure that they drink eight 8-ounce glasses of water, juice, or non-caffeinated soda a day. Remember: caffeine and alcohol work as diuretics and drain the body of water.

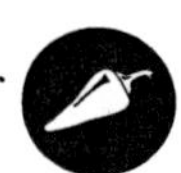

A Hot Idea

For a Class Exercise

Try this role-playing exercise.

Have one class member act as a resident who refuses to eat and another as a CNA dealing with them. Have the "resident" think of difficult residents in their care, maybe ones with dementia or other diseases, as they play their role. Have the CNA attempt to feed the "resident" and allow the class to offer suggestions.

Conduct a discussion after the role playing about which methods worked and why.

TOPIC #4

Food: The Social Significance

In addition to the nutritional importance of food, it carries social importance too. Some foods have certain cultural or religious significance. Others are associated with specific social settings and periods in a person's life. Awareness of this deeper meaning of food will help CNAs in making sure that the dining room is an atmosphere that residents can look forward to, a fun, social time, even for sick residents.

To begin, SAY:

Food is important for more than nutritional reasons. It also has an important social aspect. Mealtime is most often a time to gather with others. Some foods and meals have religious or cultural significance. Food can also evoke certain times, memories, and people. Food plays a key role in all of our lives.

As with most of us, residents associate mealtime with family time. It is a time to enjoy a well prepared meal and be with your loved ones. Ceremony and emotions are closely bound up with food. Being in a nursing facility, food can lose this sense of ceremony and special significance for a resident, and be one of the reasons for their loss of appetite. It may upset some residents to be eating food that they had no hand in preparing with people who are not family.

Think about the time before dinner in your house, the smells and the sounds of cooking, the table setting, talking with family about the upcoming meal. These start a feeling of hunger that prepares us for the meal. The body responds to these cues by sending more saliva to your mouth and digestive juices to your stomach. By the time you actually sit down to eat, you're mentally and physically ready to go. Now think about how a resident must feel. These mealtime cues are absent and they have much less control over what they eat and who they eat with. Years of eating habits they have acquired need to be changed, which can cause lots of problems.

Feeding others is one of the most loving and caring things a person can do for another. As a nursing or cooking mother, party hostess, or a CNA in a nursing home, you provide people with nourishment, as well as a sense of love and well-being. Mealtimes take on a new significance for you and the residents, when you focus on more than the nutritional aspects of food. The health, well-being, and happiness of your residents will be the reward for your caregiving.

You can help the resident by bringing back the other, non-nutritional meanings of food. Help the residents communicate at mealtime. With a little work, you will find that residents will regain their appetites, as they see food as more than just sustenance. Reintroduce them to each other to avoid embarrassment over forgotten names. Help guide the conversation to favorite foods, or foods associated with their culture or religion. You can help them anticipate the meal and the interaction, the conversation, and the genuine enjoyment of food.

DISTRIBUTE Handout 5-7: Mealtime Checklist.

Review the handout, then SAY:

This checklist deals with the practical side of a meal. As we have seen, there are other aspects. What can you do to help create atmosphere and encourage good company? Does your facility make it hard to concentrate on these non-nutritional meanings of food? How do they do this and how can you change it? What suggestions would you give them?

Have a discussion about this subject. Take appropriate class suggestions to your dietary or nursing staff. Most of all, take their suggestions seriously, since they are in the interest of the residents' well-being.

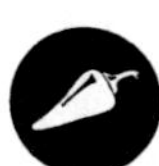

A Hot Idea

For a Class Exercise

Conduct a brainstorming session in which you ask nursing assistants to plan their ideal dinner from beginning to end.

On the board, list these categories:

- Beverages
- Soup
- Side dishes
- Appetizer
- Main course
- Dessert

Tell them to make this their dream meal, regardless of price or availability of food. Who would they invite to this meal and why?

To conclude, DISTRIBUTE Handout 5-8: QUIZ for Module 5.

Answers to the Module 5 Quiz:

1. *False*
2. *True*
3. *False*
4. *True*
5. *True*
6. *False*
7. *True*
8. *True*
9. *False*
10. *False*

MODULE 6

Spirituality and Dying

Objectives of this Module

CNAs will:

- Learn to ease the fears and anxieties that can go along with death in a nursing facility
- Appreciate residents' different spiritual needs so they can offer emotional support and understanding
- Learn the importance of mourning when a beloved resident dies

Introduction

For Instructor Only

There is a special kind of stress that comes with the job of nursing assistant — the strong emotion we call grief. Grief is real and perfectly natural. It has temporary physical symptoms which may include difficulty eating, sleeping, or carrying on with daily activities.

CNAs experience grief more often than other healthcare workers. To be a good CNA, that person has to enter fully into relationships with their residents. It follows, then, that they also acutely feel the pain of a resident's death.

Because many of us equate good caregiving with "selflessness," many CNAs may try to simply put aside their feelings of sadness or anger at the death of a resident — this can be a costly mistake.

This module focuses on helping CNAs cope with many of the issues surrounding death and dying, including spirituality of residents, caring for the dying resident, and grief and mourning.

TOPIC #1

Spirituality

Introduction — For Instructor Only

Understanding different religions and spiritualities can be a difficult aspect of a CNA's job. Some people's beliefs may seem foreign, even in opposition, to what a CNA was raised with and believes. Nonetheless, it is vitally important that, as caregivers, they learn as much as they can about different residents' religious beliefs and how they can help them practice those beliefs within the facility.

As a person grows older, they often come to rely more on their religious beliefs. In a facility with many needs to attend to, it is impossible to give each resident the perfect setting in which to practice their religious customs and rituals. As tough as it might seem, facilities are required by regulation to provide spiritual opportunities to their residents, no matter what their beliefs.

Many residents will have some spiritual affiliation or system of personal beliefs, but some may not. Though these people may not associate themselves with a particular religion, they can still have spiritual needs. Being spiritual does not have to mean adhering to a strict set of religious rules. Regardless of their visits to church or participation in ceremonies, they could still believe in a higher power.

Residents can observe their religion in various ways within the nursing facility. Some facilities are affiliated with a certain religion, which means they will emphasize that religion. Non-religiously affiliated facilities must try to aid each resident in their religious practice, whether it is traditional (such as Catholicism, Judaism, Muslim, etc.) or non-traditional (a smaller group that may be unfamiliar to staff members).

Some ways in which the facility can aid resident's religious practice are through church services, Bible or other holy book studies, and memorial ceremonies for those who have passed away in the nursing home. These memorial or remembrance ceremonies do not have to be in a particular religious context, but can greatly help the residents deal with the death of those they cared for. Services can be offered in a common room, a facility chapel, or any specially designated place. Often, clergy or other religious people are also invited to visit the residents.

To begin, SAY:

As a person ages, their spirituality can become an increasingly important part of their lives. Whatever religion or moral code they are associated with, their beliefs offer a way to focus on what is important, as well as a purpose to their suffering. In this period of their lives, with increasing thoughts of loss and death, spirituality can offer solace and strength.

How can one understand an intangible thing like spirituality? In order to define spirituality, we can start with our definition of the spirit.

As most of us agree, a human is more than just flesh and bone that lives, grows, and dies. We also think and feel. We have memories, dreams, regret, pain, and love. Our "spirit" is where these feelings lie and is what connects us to other humans. Religion, for many people, is a way to define this spirit, to give it shape, and give meaning to our existence. It also helps people understand and explain why they feel what they feel and why they're here.

Often, talking about or explaining something can help you define it or figure out your feelings toward it. As you've seen in your work with elderly residents, sometimes all they want is someone to listen to them. They want to discuss what's important to them, like their family, memories, and feelings. Your listening can help them define what's important in their lives.

Symbols, like rosary beads or a wooden cross, often help people describe what they can't communicate in words. These symbols hold deeper meaning than simply jewelry or a piece of wood. By asking a resident what these symbols mean to them, you open up a way for them to discuss their spirituality.

Sometimes, just someone to listen to them is all a resident needs. By actively listening and asking questions about their spiritual beliefs, though, you can show them that you really care. Your communication skills are key here. Listen patiently and attentively to what they have to say. If the opportunity arises, ask questions respectfully.

In your role as caregiver, you can do a lot to see that your resident's spiritual needs are met. A resident or a member of their family may specifically ask for your help. They might ask you to come to a religious service or spiritual observance. They might need your help in arranging a visit with a spiritual leader or clergyman. A physically weak or disabled resident might need help in displaying their religious items, like hanging a crucifix, putting on a yarmulke, or reading from a holy book. As we just discussed, all they may need is for you to listen to them talk about their spiritual beliefs. For some residents though, religion may be a deeply private thing, which they choose to practice alone. You must also honor that.

READ these two scenarios to the group. Have them act the scenes out, then come up with solutions to each.

1. Mrs. Snow, who has severe arthritis, is crying and frustrated because she can not hang her crucifix on her own. The CNA helps her hang it over her bed.

Something to think about: How could the CNA used this occasion to talk to Mrs. Snow about her religious beliefs?

2. Mr. Coen, a Jewish resident, asks a CNA to pray with him.

Something to think about: How can a CNA help this resident with his religious ceremony without going against his or her own beliefs?

DISTRIBUTE Handout 6-1: Religious Holidays.

Review the handout with the class. Ask the class to add anything extra they know about these holidays and if there are any holy days they would like to add to the list.

Separate the class into smaller groups, then READ them this scenario:

Mrs. Nelson is a Southern Baptist, who lived in rural Alabama her entire life. She is a loud, robust woman, who likes to sing and listen to gospel music. Mr. Klasky, a reserved Catholic man from New York, is upset by the singing and complains constantly to the CNAs. It is apparent that he is not used to Mrs. Nelson's way of expressing her spirituality.

Now have each group discuss and come up with solutions to the problem. Continue with a class discussion of everyone's answers.

TOPIC #2

The Dying Resident

One of the most trying experiences for CNAs, causing stress to both their emotional and physical health, is caring for a dying resident. Naturally, people want to try to avoid this uncomfortable topic, but it is very important for CNAs to hear and talk about it openly. If it is not discussed, CNAs are left on their own to deal with this extremely difficult situation. By openly discussing terminally ill residents, the CNA will be able to better care for them, comfort their families, and handle their own emotions.

To begin, SAY:

It isn't news to you, that, in a nursing home, people die. No one, however, should have to die terrified and alone. You can help residents die in a more peaceful and meaningful manner by offering them your support and care. There are many needs a dying resident has that you can help fulfill.

DISTRIBUTE Handout 6-2: When a Resident is Dying.

Look over and discuss the needs listed on the handout. Have CNAs tell about their experiences dealing with dying residents. Did they sense these needs? Are there any they would add to the list? How were the needs expressed and met? How did other staff and family respond to these needs?

Take Note: This is likely to be an intense and possibly emotional discussion. Take some extra time to let the CNAs talk. It might be one of the first times they have discussed this topic with so many people and so openly.

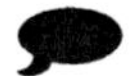

To continue, SAY:

Dr. Elisabeth Kubler-Ross in her book, *On Death and Dying,* defines five stages that a dying person goes through. Dying is a process with specific stages, like much of the rest of life. There is no strict rule that people have to follow all the stages or even experience them in order. By understanding them, though, you will be better equipped to care for dying residents. Knowing the general process can aid you in identifying the person's needs, even when they don't voice them. Good observing and listening skills will help you recognize what stage your resident might be in and to anticipate what could come next.

DISTRIBUTE Handout 6-3: The Five Stages of Dying.

After reading Kubler-Ross's five stages aloud, ask the class if they have any questions. Can they give examples from their experience of the stages? Also make a point of focusing on any CNAs who currently have a dying resident in their care.

Then SAY:

Your own feelings about death can have a big impact on how you handle a dying resident. If you find the topic hard to discuss, you might not be able to talk to a dying resident about their situation or to other residents when another resident passes away. Fear of death may cause you to avoid dying residents. If a resident's dying is upsetting to you, you may unintentionally treat a dying resident as if they were no longer a living person.

People often avoid talking about death and dying altogether, which makes it hard to deal with a dying resident who wants to talk about their situation. Nursing home staffs usually become much closer with their patients than staff in other healthcare settings. This closeness can lead to feelings of grief, helplessness, frustration, or anger when a resident dies.

In some cultures, discussing death or touching a dead body is taboo and socially unacceptable. If we know about their customs and views of death, we can respond to those individuals appropriately. If at all possible, find out these things about the resident ahead of time.

It is crucial that we discuss our personal feelings about death and dying with our residents, and each other. If we can openly express these feelings, we can more easily help ourselves, each other, and our dying residents.

Since personal reservations and fears about death can have such an impact on your care for a dying resident, you should clarify your feelings about death and dying. Here are some questions to help you define your feelings.

DISTRIBUTE Handout 6-4: Your Beliefs.

Ask your class to privately think about and answer these questions. The goal here is to understand our own feelings, thoughts, and beliefs regarding death and dying. Once the class has had an opportunity to write their responses, see if anyone would be willing to share theirs.

TOPIC #3

Grief and Mourning

Introduction — For Instructor Only

The best CNAs enter completely and emotionally into relationships with their residents. For this reason, grief hits them more often than most any other healthcare worker. Coping with the intense pain of a favorite resident's death requires a lot of time and understanding from others.

Researchers say that if a CNA has not grieved fully over the loss of a favorite resident, they are more likely to experience burn-out and leave their job. In their personal interest, and in the interest of reducing turnover in your facility, helping CNAs cope with grief is extremely important.

Some CNAs may think that being a good caregiver means never thinking of themselves. This could not be further from the truth. If they are emotionally burned out, they will become increasingly less effective as caregivers.

Our society often makes grieving an even more difficult process than it already is. Grieving is completely natural and normal when a loved one is lost. Experts say that grieving is the best way to recover from a death.

A grieving person often can't eat, sleep, or perform their daily activities. Its strictly physical symptoms can last from twenty minutes to an hour or longer. Each person's grieving technique is distinct. It is imperative that CNAs be given adequate time for their grieving process and not immediately be forced back to their daily work demands.

To begin, SAY:

Grief is natural and necessary. It is not just a response to loss, but a method for recovering from that loss. There are temporary physical symptoms. You may have trouble eating, sleeping, or fulfilling your daily activities. The most natural response to the loss, though, is crying.

If you are grieving in a healthy environment, tears don't bring shame; they are understood as the natural way to release feelings of sadness. Tears, as well as often making one feel emotionally better, have been proved to make you feel physically better, by releasing toxins from your body.

There is a prejudice that everyone should grieve in the same way, cry the proper amount of time, and act in a certain manner. In fact, everyone grieves in their own unique way. No one should or can judge the depth of another's grief from their exterior appearance.

It should be noted that here is a type of grief called "anticipatory grief," which can begin before the person has died. It prepares you for a dying loved one's unavoidable death, and for the feelings that will come after death. Time must be allowed for this kind of grief, as it better prepares a person for the intense emotions that will follow the death.

Have a discussion where CNAs are free to define grief in their own words and let them write their responses on the board. Remind them that each person grieves in their own way and in their own good time. Also stress that grieving is a natural response that can be expressed in healthy and unhealthy ways. Use these questions to guide their answers:

- *Which emotions are involved in grieving?*
- *In addition to sadness, can guilt and anger be part of grief?*
- *List several healthy and, conversely, unhealthy ways to express your grief.*

DISTRIBUTE Handout 6-5: The Stages of Grief.

Review the handout with the class and compare it to what they have come up with on their own.

Then SAY:

Grief is never an easy process, but it is a normal one. Everyone has their own way and amount of time in which to do it. The pain of this period is critical for helping you through this emotional time.

Society often considers discussion of death as morbid or something you just can't talk about. Even in a nursing home where it is a regular reality, people often keep the subject hush hush. Seeing another's grief reminds people of the reality of death, which most people prefer to forget. People need to get past this idea, because someone who is grieving needs support and care, not avoidance and feelings of anxiousness from others.

In the past, mourning had a set period of time and the grieving person was treated with special care. They mostly wore black to express their emotional state. Today, things are not as formal, and often people do not show the same concern. A grieving person needs others to acknowledge their pain and to be understanding, or the pain can worsen.

Grieving is a difficult process, but it can't be avoided if one wants to recover from a loss. Not expressing your sadness and anger will only prolong the mourning. Failure to deal with the emotional pain can lead to depression, burn-out, and other stress-related illnesses.

As you've seen, intense emotions accompany grief. You must be patient and understanding with a grieving person as they go through these feelings. You will probably need their support one day. Being compassionate to the grieving person will help foster an open environment where death and grief can be discussed. It is an unavoidable part of working in a nursing home and the more the pain can be shared and eased, the better.

You are the direct caregivers for many people and see more death and dying than in most other professions. Also, you are often personally close to the residents that you work with. Because of these job realities, CNAs need to show strength and support for one another. If you know a co-worker has recently lost a favorite resident, help them by acknowledging their pain. Offer them comfort and be understanding if their work is not totally up to par.

A phone call, a card, or a little note is a wonderful gesture to show then someone's thinking about them. Offering to listen to them or even giving a simple hug can help immeasurably. Acknowledge the close relationship they had with the deceased and reassure them that they will recover from the loss and that you will be there to help them. And always, let the person know that it's okay to show their grief.

Now ask the class to think about a time when they lost a loved one. Have them recall what those around them did to help them through their mourning. What specific things were most helpful?

End this module by reminding the class about your facility's resources for CNAs who are grieving over the loss of a resident. Let them know if time is allowed off for funerals. Also, be sure to give them information on bereavement counseling or other help they can seek, if they wish.

To conclude, DISTRIBUTE Handout 6-6: QUIZ for Module 6.

Answers to the Module 6 Quiz:

1. True	*6. False*
2. False	*7. True*
3. True	*8. True*
4. False	*9. True*
5. False	*10. False*

MODULE 7

Your Residents' Quality of Life

Objectives of this Module

CNAs will:

- Outline ways to make new residents feel at home
- Learn the need to understand and empathize with their residents
- Foster the residents' independence while committing to a defense of their rights
- Be alert to the signs of psychosocial difficulties, especially depression

Introduction

For Instructor Only

Who has a greater impact on residents' quality of life than nursing assistants? According to a recent Consumer Reports article about life in America's nursing homes, nursing assistants provide 90 percent of the direct care residents receive. These days, that means providing care to residents who are generally older, more frail, medically unstable, and often cognitively impaired.

In such a caregiving environment, it becomes paramount that the nursing assistant understand the needs, desires, and rights of the residents to ensure the best possible care. Therefore, this module focuses on helping CNAs develop empathy and understanding around such issues as resident independence, new residents, residents' rights, and the psychosocial issues that come with being a resident in a nursing home.

TOPIC #1

Welcoming the New Resident

To begin, SAY:

Pretend that you are 80 years old and you've just been told that you have to move into a nursing home. You've lived independently, since your spouse died 15 years ago. You have a large house that you've tried to take care of by yourself. Your kids try to tell you the nursing home is nice, that you will be with people like yourself, that it's for your own good. You begin to wonder what you can bring with you, what you will be allowed to do, and what things in your life will change.

DISTRIBUTE Handout 7-1: The New Resident.

Then SAY:

See how difficult that was to do? This is similar to what most of your new residents are faced with when they move into our facility. New residents often feel vulnerable, fearful, disoriented, even abandoned and hopeless, and who can blame them? As a CNA, since you will be working most closely with the resident, how can you help them through this difficult time?

A new resident's recent life has often been full of pain and loss, sometimes involving the deaths of close family, friends, or spouse. The move into a long term care facility is more than a move to a new house. They are giving up many possessions, maybe their home, but worst of all, their independence. As you saw in the handout, the new resident loses the ability to choose. Not being able to sit in an easy chair anymore may seem minor, but to a new resident, it represents a lot more. It represents a loss of choice.

The best thing you can do is get to know the new resident as a real person. What are their likes? Dislikes? What was their life like before the facility? Viewing them as an individual will make this big transition much easier for them.

Ask the class to come up with a list of ways that they can get to know the new resident. What are the most important things to learn about them? Write their answers on the board and add the ones listed below, if they are not mentioned:

- *What kinds of things do they like to do?*
- *Is/Was the resident married?*
- *Do they have children? Grandchildren?*
- *Did they have a career or job?*
- *What are their fears?*
- *Do they have religious beliefs?*
- *What do they enjoy doing?*
- *What things or people make them very happy?*

Review the list on the board. Ask for ways that your class could get the answers to these questions. Do they ask the resident directly? Do they ask a family member? Do they look for photos or special objects that could offer clues?

To continue, SAY:

What things are being achieved in this "getting to know you" period? Mainly, you are making the resident and family more comfortable and showing you value that resident as more than a resident, but as an individual. What you learn from the resident and family in this period will help you with the resident's adjustment process. Remember, what you do in the first few days and weeks will help build a lasting close relationship with the resident and their family.

DISTRIBUTE Handout 7-2: New Resident Tipsheet.

Review the handout with the class.

DISTRIBUTE Handout 7-3: Meeting the New Resident.

Ask three class members to volunteer in this role-playing exercise. One will play the resident, one the family member, and the other the CNA. The rest of the class should watch, comment, and coach the players.

Now have a group discussion as scripted below. Ask the players the following questions and allow for comments from the class.

Now SAY:

Of course, in real life, you have more time to make the resident feel comfortable in their new home. Your first impression can leave a lasting impression on family members and residents alike. Your relations with them in the future may depend on how comfortable they initially feel with you. So, try to go out of your way to make them feel welcome in this new and foreign place.

"Resident": Did the CNA make you feel welcome? Did you feel frightened? Confused? What would have made you feel more comfortable?

"Family member": Did you feel that the CNA took your concern for your parent seriously? What was your first impression of the staff through his CNA? What did they do to make you feel comfortable about your decision to put your loved one in this facility?

"CNA": What did this first meeting tell you about the new resident? What did it tell you about their family? What did you do to make the resident and family member feel more comfortable? How involved do you think this family member will be? Did you show them you were interested in them as an individual?

Ask the class: Did the CNA do a good job at making the resident and their family member comfortable? What else could they have done to put them at ease? Also, ask participants if they can recall a difficult admission. How it was handled? Could it have been improved upon?

To continue, SAY:

How can an unknown place, full of unknown people be home? Home is not a specific house or town — it's a feeling of comfort, safety, and belonging. Your goal is to help the new resident feel that the facility is safe and comfortable. As they begin to feel more comfortable in their new surroundings and make friends, the new resident may be able to start thinking of the facility as home.

Your main goal should be familiarizing the resident with their surroundings and their new routine. You should also help them form friendships with other residents, as well as yourself. In this time, they may feel overwhelmed and beg to go home. As a compassionate CNA, you will resist the urge to tell them the facility "is now their home."

Helping a new resident recapture their sense of individuality is probably the most important thing you can do. Making an extra effort to know the resident as an individual will help them feel safe. Some CNAs say that a new resident starts to feel adjusted when they start complaining. This means they have gained enough confidence, and comfort with you, to voice their opinion.

Unfortunately, some people think the family should stay away during this period, so that the new resident will wake up to the reality of their situation more quickly. This could not be more wrong. The new resident and their family especially need each other during this difficult period of adjustment. The family may be confused or guilty about their decision to put a loved one in a nursing facility. The resident may feel upset and alone. Your job as a CNA is to make both sides more comfortable, which will ease the adjustment for everyone.

STOP **TAKE A BREAK.**

TOPIC #2

Distress and Depression

 **To begin, SAY:**

The majority of us feel positive about ourselves and the people around us. Most of us like our jobs and our family and community roles. We hope that this positive self-image will last into our later years and, usually, it will. Things can change drastically, though. We can lose the people we love. We can lose our liveliness, what made us want to wake up in the morning. We all age in different ways and, as we change, our social and emotional needs change, too.

Aging is normal and universal. It affects each of us differently. Inevitable changes in health and relationships will affect people differently. Some elderly people stay active, healthy, and social. Many others, though, fall ill and experience a series of losses. Physical problems start increasing. Spouses, family, or friends may die. Children and grandchildren may live far away or lead hectic lives. These changes can leave an elderly person feeling desolate and depressed. Life conditions such as these, and often others in addition, put elderly people living in nursing facilities at an extremely high risk for psychosocial problems.

Let's think about our residents for a moment and ask ourselves: What are their basic psychological and social needs?

Encourage your class to share what the basic psychosocial needs of their residents are. Write the answers on the board and allow for discussion. Use the following list as a guideline for discussion:

- *friendship*
- *recreation*
- *respect*
- *the feeling of being needed*
- *sexuality*
- *touch*
- *meaningful activity*
- *spirituality*
- *independence*

DISTRIBUTE Handout 7-4: Causes of Psychosocial Distress.

Have the class look over the handout, as you read it aloud. Ask them for ideas of ways they can counteract these causes. How can they make the resident feel less isolated? How can they help adjust them to new roles?

DISTRIBUTE Handout 7-5: Common Signs of Depression.

Then SAY:

A resident with untreated depression may see a bleak life in front of them. If you know the common symptoms of depression, you will be able to alert someone who can help early on, saving the resident unnecessary suffering. Your understanding and comfort can help a resident overcome this terrible emotional pain.

Depression has physical and emotional effects, and it is sometimes referred to as a whole body disorder. It can lead to confusion, memory loss, and poor judgement, as well as unexplained aches and pains. It may be mistaken for dementia or Alzheimer's. Worst of all, it can take away a person's will to live.

The good news is that, with the right treatment, the symptoms of clinical depression almost always improve, sometimes within just a few weeks. The bad news is that often, in nursing facilities, residents don't get the treatment they need because their caregivers think that their symptoms are just a part of getting old. In fact, it is estimated that more than 30 percent of nursing home residents are depressed, but of that 30 percent, only 30 percent are ever diagnosed and treated. That is a lot of unnecessary suffering.

Depression comes in two forms: major depression and bipolar disorder. Major depression makes normal life almost impossible to live. It takes away pleasure and meaning from life. The other, bipolar disorder, is sometimes referred to as manic-depressive illness. It consists of severe mood swings that alternate from high to low. While in the depressive phase, a person is so low they can barely function. They may even be suicidal. While in the manic phase, a person's mind races and they often have sleep problems. Agitation and pacing may also be a part of the manic phase.

WRITE on the board:

- Grief
- Genetics
- Personality
- Medications
- Other illnesses

Then SAY:

Among elderly people, some of the common causes of depression are:

Grief. Sadness is a normal response to loss, and elderly people in nursing facilities have usually lost a great deal. When symptoms of depression last for long periods of time, a professional assessment should be done.

Genetics. Clinical depression runs in families. Those with depression in their family are particularly vulnerable.

Personality. Low self-esteem and over-dependence on others can make people more susceptible to depression.

Medications. Some medicines have depressive side-effects, especially drugs used to treat high blood pressure (hypertension) and arthritis.

Other illnesses. Stroke, some cancers, diabetes, Parkinson's disease, and hormonal disorders can cause clinical depression. People with dementia can also suffer from clinical depression. Anything that affects the brain chemistry can cause clinical depression.

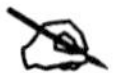

WRITE on the board:

- Psychotherapy
- Medication
- Electro-convulsive therapy (ECT)

Then SAY:

Clinical depression has three major treatments: psychotherapy, medication, and electro-convulsive therapy (ECT).

1. **Psychotherapy.** Talking with a trained therapist can be very effective for some people in treating clinical depression. Sometimes it is used in combination with medication.

2. **Medication.** Medications alter the movement of brain chemicals, improving mood, sleep, appetite, concentration, and energy level. People react differently to different medications. With the right medication and the right dose, improvement can be seen quickly.

3. Electro-convulsive therapy (ECT). A very carefully administered, brief dose of electricity can be an effective treatment for severe depression. It can also be used for a person who cannot tolerate medications or their side-effects.

To sum up, depression's effects are particularly harsh on the elderly. Though symptoms can be different from person to person, they all have serious emotional and physical implications. Depression makes people susceptible to many other illnesses, as it weakens the body. A depressed resident may appear to have dementia, but this is really pseudo-dementia, or false dementia. Depression can be so awful that, if untreated, people sometimes take their own lives. By knowing the signs of depression and taking immediate action, you can help ease suffering and even help save a life.

Have you had any residents with depression? What signs did they give of the illness? How were they treated? What did you do to help them?

TOPIC #3

Residents' Independence

 **To begin, SAY:**

Think about your daily routine. What do you do when you wake up? Do you immediately go for a cup of coffee or do you like to lay in bed for 15 minutes after your alarm? Do you spend time in the morning in front of your TV or on the phone with friends? Maybe you like to take a long shower or do some stretches to warm up for the upcoming day. Maybe you do your grocery shopping before work, maybe after work. You can decide whether to make your lunch or stop by a favorite restaurant. Your day is made up of endless choices, choices that you have the freedom to make for yourself.

The independence you require to make all the little daily decisions may seem unimportant to you now. It is a part of your life that you can take for granted, as a physically active, independent adult. The routine may even seem boring to you, but remember, it's made up of choices you've made. You can change it whenever you please. The freedom to control your life, to make your own choices, is called autonomy and is something many residents sacrifice when they move into a nursing facility.

ASK the group these questions and write their answers on the board.

- How many choices can our residents make in their day to day routine?
- Can they eat whenever they please?
- Do they decide when they want visitors?
- Can they choose their own activities?
- Are they free to decorate their rooms however they want?

To continue, SAY:

Think about how you, as a CNA, can promote a resident's independence. Think about the particular ways you can help.

TAKE NOTE: It would be useful here to have your facility's policies on residents' rights. Review them with the class as you discuss the following areas.

SAY:

1. Schedules.

How much flexibility can you allow your residents without making your duties too difficult? Do you have to attend to that person at that specific time? Ask your residents what schedule they would ideally like to have and try to work your schedule around it. Maybe you can switch your order of activities to offer the residents more options.

2. Opportunities for contribution.

Having responsibilities, even very small ones, can help residents feel more comfortable and happy in the nursing facility. Think back to our discussion on psychosocial needs. Feeling needed is essential to a resident. Having a daily chore, a plant, even a pet if they're allowed, will give them a sense of purpose and usefulness.

3. Residents' rooms.

Everyone needs their own space, and we all have certain ways of making a space our own. Using decorations, pictures, special objects, and furniture, we design a place where we feel safe and comfortable. Let the residents have as much say in designing their space, as possible. As long as their decorating will not put anyone in danger, let them do it. It fulfills a deeper emotional need than simply beautifying.

4. Residents with dementia.

It can be much harder to foster independence in a resident with dementia. It is important to know and respect their preferences, even if they can't express them as clearly as others. A demented resident's family, as well as staff who know them well, can help you figure out their wishes before the illness. Demented residents also have the right to control their life through the choices they make.

TOPIC #4

Residents' Rights

 **To begin, SAY:**

Rules almost always have a purpose or goal behind them. The Resident Bill of Rights, which you will see in any nursing facility, reminds us that residents have rights too. The goal of these rules is to make sure residents' humanity is respected and honored, even if they may be weak, injured, or ill.

In your role as CNA, you can help protect your resident's rights. You know their needs and wishes, since you work so closely with them. You can defend their rights and help give them a better quality of life.

You are the protector and defender of their rights. Protect them from others who challenge their independence, pride, or privacy. Treat them the way they want to be treated and give them the respect they deserve.

Make sure your class knows what an ***ombudsman*** *is. In brief, an ombudsman is someone who acts as an advocate for the rights of residents in nursing and rest homes as part of a state and federally mandated program. An ombudsman receives, investigates, and tries to resolve complaints regarding resident care or quality of life.*

 **DISTRIBUTE Handout 7-6: Remember R.A.P.I.D.**

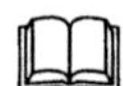 **READ the handout aloud to the class.**

To conclude, DISTRIBUTE Handout 7-7: QUIZ for Module 7.

Answers to the Module 7 Quiz:

1. *False*
2. *True*
3. *False*
4. *False*
5. *False*
6. *False*
7. *True*
8. *False*
9. *True*
10. *True*

MODULE 8

Dementia Care

Objectives of this Module

CNAs will:

- Outline the fundamentals of what constitutes dementia
- Learn a practical approach for handling problem behaviors associated with dementia
- Look at difficult behaviors as a form of communication

Introduction

For Instructor Only

This module focuses on giving your class participants a deeper understanding of dementia. They will also gain the knowledge necessary to first manage the aggressive behavior often associated with dementia, and then understand how to interpret those behaviors to discover what difficulties the resident might be having.

A recent study found that in just 25 years, there may be as many as 22 million people suffering from Alzheimer's. Already, dealing with the dementia related to the disease, as well as other kinds of dementia, makes up a significant portion of the CNAs work life.

TAKE NOTE: For this topic, it may be helpful to bring in someone from your facility to answer questions about dementia and Alzheimer's. Also, make sure to refresh your knowledge on the subject.

TOPIC #1

Understanding Dementia

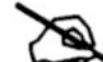

To begin, WRITE the following on the board:

Some of the behaviors most commonly associated with dementia are:

- wandering
- hitting
- verbal aggression
- screaming

Ask the class to come up with other behaviors that they associate with dementia. Make sure the following are listed:

- *mistaking someone for another person*
- *paranoia*
- *inability to sleep*
- *suspicion*
- *inappropriate sexual behavior*
- *thinking it is a past time*

Have the class discuss the list. Ask them which behaviors they think are the most difficult and why.

To continue, SAY:

To manage the difficult behaviors of dementia, you should first know why they happen. Let's take the following quiz and see how much you know about the subject.

DISTRIBUTE Handout 8-1: Dementia Quiz.

Then SAY:

Let's look at a definition of dementia, before we look at the correct answers to the quiz.

DISTRIBUTE Handout 8-2: Dementia Defined.

The correct answer to every question on the quiz is false. Now discuss the answers with the class.

SAY:

1. Dementia is only caused by Alzheimer's.

False. Dementia can also be caused by things like strokes and medication problems, as well as HIV and other viruses. If a person with dementia is properly treated by a physician, they can sometimes get rid of other causes and help improve their health.

2. Alzheimer's has a cure.

False. Nobody knows what causes Alzheimer's disease, so there are no cures. Hopefully, as research continues, a cure will be found.

3. Dementia is a natural part of growing old.

False. People often have trouble with their memory as they get older, but dementia is more severe than this. People with dementia lose the ability to reason, think, and learn.

4. Alzheimer's runs in families.

False. There is a slightly larger chance that if someone in your immediate family suffered from Alzheimer's, then you will get it. For the most part, family members of demented patients do not get dementia.

5. New changes and challenges are good for someone with severe dementia.

False. People with severe dementia need a calm, reliable environment. When changes occur often, they can become scared or agitated.

6. People with dementia act up on purpose to bother you.

False. Social abilities are affected by dementia and can make people act drastically different from their normal demeanor. They often have minimal control over their behavior.

7. Since dementia is contagious, you can catch it from a resident.

False. Dementia is not contagious.

TOPIC #2

Managing Problem Behaviors

To begin, SAY:

A resident who screams incessantly, attacks you, cries for her dead husband, and tries to get out of the facility is reacting to something in her inner or outer environment. Your job is to figure out what she is responding to and how you can help her. Remember, as strange or scary as her behavior gets, it is not personally directed towards you. The resident is reacting to her experience, not to you.

Now, let's look specifically at three of the difficult behaviors and their causes, as well as tips for you to help deal with them.

WRITE on the board:

1. Wandering

Then SAY:

We all know what it's like to chase a wandering resident and to lead them back to their room over and over again. We have all had to respond to alarms set off by residents.

Their wandering may appear to have no purpose, but it does. Often, demented residents cannot tell us why they wander, but there are ways for you to figure it out. Some reasons that residents wander are:

Short-term memory loss

A resident may start going to a destination, then forget where they were going. Ask them how they feel and try to figure out where they could have been headed. Did they need to use the bathroom? Were they hungry?

Fear

A demented resident will often wander to get away from something that they are afraid of. Even if you can't figure out where the fear comes from, reassure them and make them feel safe. Try to focus their attention somewhere else, to distract them from the fear.

Boredom

A resident may simply need stimulation to keep them from getting restless. Keep them involved with people and activities that will interest them.

Researchers have found that often residents who open doors are not trying to leave. They can be attracted by the shiny brass bars or knobs on the door. Try covering the bar with a cloth and watch how many fewer alarms are set off. Curiosity may also be a reason for residents to open doors which have windows. Shut the shade or blind on the door to keep them from opening the door in curiosity.

To continue, SAY:

How do you deal with wandering residents? Are there any little tricks that have worked for you?

There is one useful approach called validation or "therapeutic fibbing." This approach suggests you go along with a demented residents' delusions. If they believe they must be in a certain place, validate their belief and play along. Then try to focus their attention somewhere else.

Think of a resident who believes they must go to the grocery store to prepare for a big dinner. You may want to simply bring them back to their room and ignore their false belief. This could lead the resident to become agitated, which, in turn, will be stressful for you. Ignoring and refusing them may make them more determined to accomplish their imaginary task. They may feel persecuted by you for denying them what they need to do.

Some fast thinking and talking is needed here. In this example, you could offer to do the resident's shopping for them. Tell them you will go to the market after work. Ask them to make up a grocery list and ask where they usually like to go shopping.

"Therapeutic fibbing" can turn a potentially upsetting situation into a good one. Their anxiety will be relieved and you will feel better knowing you helped soothe them. Think of it as improvising or acting, which might also make it a little more fun for you.

A Hot Idea

For a Class Exercise

Try a "therapeutic fibbing" exercise with the class. Have one class member play a demented resident and one class member play a CNA. Have the "resident" head for the door and the CNA try to stop them. Have the "resident" use one of the following excuses:

- I need to go to my car. It's right outside.
- They're chasing me again! I have to leave.
- I need to get to work.

The goal is for the CNA to stop the "resident" from getting out the door, by using "therapeutic fibbing." Have the class help out the CNA if they can't convince the "resident." Have various class members play the two roles, until all the scenarios have been acted out.

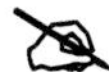

WRITE on the board:

2. Screaming

Then SAY:

Screaming can be extremely difficult for those around a demented resident. Always look for a possible cause of pain, as a demented resident will often be unable to communicate their pain.

Screaming could also be a response to a more simple discomfort, like a sensory overload or not enough sensory stimulation. Change the noise in their environment, either getting rid of extra noise or playing music. Offer them something to do, if you sense that they are bored.

Ask the class if they have any suggestions to keep a screaming resident calm.

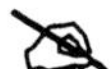

WRITE:

3. Aggression

SAY:

The third difficult behavior is aggression. There are various reasons for a resident to become angry or aggressive, such as their physical condition, life experiences, and the environment around them.

Physical conditions

Dementia can cause physical and verbal outbursts, especially for residents with some mental impairment. A brain injury, as well, can cause a person to act aggressively.

Life experience

Some of your residents may have a history of violent behavior. In the past, their way of dealing with anger could have been aggression and violence, which they have carried into the nursing facility.

Environmental factors

If a resident feels frustrated with the environment or situation, they may act out aggressively. It may occur during dressing, feeding, or bathing, as many residents get frustrated and confused by these activities.

Always keep in mind that unless you've done something deliberately to provoke a resident, then you are not personally responsible for the anger they feel or the aggression they express.

DISTRIBUTE Handout 8-3: I.C.R.P.

(Note: Handout 8-3 is four pages long.)

To continue, SAY:

What I'm giving you now is a four-step approach to anger and aggression in residents. We call it I.C.R.P. — Identify, Calm, Resolve, Prevent. This is the ICRP approach, and what we want to do here is to make this approach second nature for you. We want to think "I.C.R.P!" whenever we have to deal with an aggressive outburst from a resident. If you train yourself to use this approach, you will be less likely to get caught in the resident's negativity, and better able to do whatever can be done to help the situation.

After discussing the handout with the class, have them each remember a situation where a resident became aggressive or violent. Have them tell their stories and how they resolved the problems. Have them, with help from the class, come up with an I-C-R-P for their remembered experience.

TOPIC #3

Staying Safe

 **To begin, SAY:**

There is no way to eliminate all of a resident's anger, but you can keep yourself safe from injury. The trick is to know when an angry resident is becoming aggressive and how to prevent this. Keep these factors in mind, when dealing with an aggressive resident:

Distance

Always give an angry resident the room you think they need. Getting too close to an angry resident will only worsen a situation. If you approach them, they may feel threatened and try to strike out at you to keep you away.

Voice tone and volume

Keep your tone non-threatening and calm. If a resident is screaming or shouting, your shouting back will only make things worse.

Body posture and touch

You may want to offer the resident a reassuring gesture, like placing a hand on their shoulder or hugging them. They may see this as a threat or an attack and respond accordingly. Never touch an angry resident. Monitor your posture and position, as well. Keep eye level with them, try to keep from stiffening or tensing up your body, and never point. These body movements may just incite more anger.

Be flexible

If you think the resident is angry about a task you are performing, put the task on hold and allow time for their anger to go away. They are often frustrated or angry over their loss of control and may react against you. Give them choices about when and how you will perform the task.

Get help

As we saw with the ICRP approach, maybe you are not the best person to help a particular resident. Getting their favorite CNA may calm them down. Also, never be afraid to ask for help when a resident is aggressive with you and you can't handle it alone.

Have a discussion about everything you've learned in this module. Tell the class that you understand these behaviors can be disturbing and hard to deal with. Then, have them discuss the emotions these behaviors cause in them. Bring up the fact that suppressing your anger or hurt, and trying to always be professional can have negative consequences. The emotions could surface later. Encourage them to suggest ways to prevent this from happening.

To end, tell the class that they need to support one another in these situations. Have them all find a fellow staff member with whom they can discuss the emotions that aggressive residents bring up in them.

To conclude, DISTRIBUTE Handout 8-4: QUIZ for Module 8.

Answers to the Module 8 Quiz:

1. False	*6. False*
2. False	*7. False*
3. False	*8. False*
4. True	*9. True*
5. True	*10. True.*

MODULE 9

The Importance of Family

Objectives of this Module

CNAs will:

- Learn that they must work together with family members to achieve the best care for the resident
- Gain new insight into family members' occasionally frustrating behavior
- Be empowered to act calmly and professionally in stressful situations with residents' families

Introduction

For Instructor Only

One of the most important and potentially most volatile relationships in a long term care facility is between family members and CNAs. These interactions can cause major stress. It is essential that this relationship run smoothly to ensure the quality of the resident's care.

Sometimes, CNAs feel that the family blames them for things that they have little or no control over, which can lead to anger and frustration. Conflict management techniques, listening skills, and problem-solving strategies can help reduce CNA stress and help them foster strong, understanding relationships with residents' families.

TOPIC #1

Caring Together: Family and Staff

To begin, SAY:

Everyone benefits — and especially the resident — when CNAs and families work well together. But sometimes it can be hard. On one hand, the family wants to be assured that their relative is receiving good care. On the other, CNAs can offer care more effectively when families cooperate and inform them about a resident's special needs.

Open communication with the resident's family can help the CNA to know the resident as an individual, instead of just another patient. The information they have to offer about their relative's past life is invaluable and something only they can give; Maybe he was a fine carpenter or maybe she loved to garden.

An idea for personalizing your facility and its care is to encourage families to create a bulletin board or scrapbook with information about their loved ones. It can contain anything that will let staff (and other residents) know about the resident's history: photos, awards, diplomas — whatever highlights the resident's personality. It's a great way to share information about who the resident was before the nursing home. It can also work as a conversation starter between family and staff.

Ask the group for some other suggestions on making residents more comfortable, things from their real life experience as CNAs.

To continue, SAY:

Of course family members care about the quality of their loved one's care. But one sociologist, who talked to numerous residents' relatives, found that they were more concerned that the CNAs really cared about their relatives as individuals.

With some very simple gestures, you can let the family know that you really do care. Make sure to talk to them when they visit their relative. Tell them what their loved one does every day and about things you've discovered — what they like to do and what music they like. These small acts tell relatives that you are giving attention to their loved one and thinking of him or her as a real person, which in turn makes them feel more secure about leaving their loved one in your care.

As simple as this may seem, family-staff relations can still be extremely difficult.

DISTRIBUTE Handout 9-1: How the Family Fits In.

SAY:

Experts believe that a nursing home can be viewed as a whole made up of three interlocking parts: the residents, the family, and the staff. Since these three parts interlock, a problem in one will affect all the others, thus affecting the whole system.

So, if there are problems among the residents, then staff and family will feel the stress. If there is a problem with the staff, then residents and family members will both be affected by it, too. If family members are acting inappropriately or disagreeing with one another, then staff and residents will also feel the strain. The wellness of the whole depends on the wellness of each part.

This interlocking model is not a method for laying blame, but simply a way to understand how the relationships between these three groups work. Think of an Alzheimer's patient and the effect their disease has on the staff and family. The disease is no fault of the resident's, yet it still has repercussions with the other two groups.

Looking at the diagram, do you think this model is true? Can you think of any examples to illustrate it?

It is important to maintain good bonds between residents and family for many reasons. Primarily, their visits keep the resident feeling comfortable, oriented, and loved.

Keeping up a relationship with the resident is important for the families, too. Family history is an important part of family life, which should not be lost. The resident's relative needs this connection with their elder as much as the resident needs the connection to their family to feel complete. As a CNA, you can nurture this relationship.

TOPIC #2

The Family's Point of View

 **To begin, SAY:**

Often, families feel guilty about deciding to place a relative in a nursing home. They could have split emotions about their decision — feeling both relieved and anxious at once. Putting a loved one in someone else's care is always a difficult choice.

You can try to help the family feel that they've made a good decision. It will help if they feel assured that their relative is getting quality, individualized care. Some may fear that their loved one is being neglected. As caregivers, we know this is unfounded, but it is still a fear for the family.

If you are having problems or conflicts with family members, keep their confused feelings in mind; it could help you have sympathy for their position. They may mis-direct their anger at you, since you are now the one closest to their relatives. Your best option to ease any negative feelings is in trying to connect with the family. By showing them warmth and concern, they will be reassured that their relative is receiving the same care that you've shown them.

A positive relationship between you and the family member is crucial to the resident having a good experience in the facility. In the big picture, concern shown for the family is concern shown to the resident. So building a good relationship with the family is time well spent.

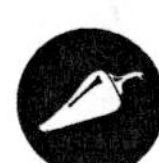

A Hot Idea

For a Class Exercise

Have each member of the class write down a specific way that they have helped improve communication with family members and encouraged the family member's involvement with their loved one's care. Ask them also to write down what their single greatest challenge in working with residents' families has been.

Draw a vertical line on your chalk board and label one column + (a positive) and the other – (a negative). Ask the group to share what they've written, listing their remarks in the appropriate column. When everyone has finished, review and discuss the items in each column.

Note: Occasionally, nursing home policy can be a roadblock to good communication with families. If this is true in your facility, you may decide as a group how to constructively bring these problems to the attention of your administration.

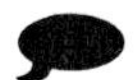

To continue, SAY:

When family members are arguing due to different expectations for a resident's care, things can get very sticky. You can politely tell them that it's very difficult for the staff when the family doesn't speak with a unified voice. When this happens, try to sit down together with the social worker to come to an agreement. A caregiver should not have to face this issue alone.

At times, family doesn't understand the care needs of their loved one and asks for things contrary to your facility's care plan. Again, a nurse or social worker would be helpful here to explain the care-planning team's side of the situation.

Family members may ask the staff members questions that they're not equipped to answer. It's okay for you to not have all the answers and better that you don't answer incorrectly. So, don't hesitate to re-direct a question that you are unsure of to the proper department.

Here's an example of a stressful family-staff interaction.

READ this aloud to the class:

Mr. Thomas is in the late stages of Alzheimer's and in poor physical condition. He cannot recognize staff or family members and feels suspicious of both. He refuses to take medicine and, more often lately, food from them.

His daughter, Teresa, is extremely upset and believes that the facility should force her father to eat and take his medicine. She fears he might die without nutrition or medicine, and threatens to blame the staff if this should happen. Her brother, Dennis, has been chosen by their father to act as his medical treatment guardian. He, too, is distressed about the situation, but constantly reminds her that they must obey their father's wishes.

Brother and sister argue continually when they visit the facility. Teresa wants to take action, ignoring her father's wishes, and force feed him manually or through an I.V. "It's the disease, it's not Dad acting," she says. Dennis stands by his father's wish not to be forced physically to eat or take medicine: "Dad always said that if he became extremely ill, he did not want to be forced to eat against his will. We have to respect his wish."

Who do you side with? Why?

TOPIC #3

Resolving Family Conflict

To begin, DISTRIBUTE Handout 9-2: Conflict Resolution.

While the class is reviewing the handout, SAY:

CNAs, especially those who have been on the job a long time, understand that positive relations with residents' families are essential to providing quality care for their residents. Veteran CNAs understand that, for family members, placing a relative in a nursing facility can be very stressful. Family members can mistakenly aim their confused feelings at the CNA by criticizing and accusing. If you fully understand the steps outlined in this handout, you will be more equipped to resolve conflict with family members.

1. Have the person thoroughly explain their complaint.

Hear the person out fully before you jump on the defensive. You may feel frustration and want to block them out. Take a deep breath and listen openly. Their opinion and information are key factors in reaching a solution.

2. Be clear that you understand their complaint.

After you hear them out completely, repeat what they've said back to them. This should immediately diffuse some of the heated feelings around the subject. It will show them that you are open to their side and understand what they are saying. You don't have to agree, merely understand.

3. Look for the need or reason behind the problem.

Understand that the family member's high emotions, even the negative ones, stem out of love for the resident. A complaint about an apparently minor issue could represent a deeper emotion, such as anger, fear, or guilt, about their loved one's position. By not brushing off their complaint as meaningless, you help reassure their troubled feelings. An acknowledgement of their love and concern for the resident could make you and the family member feel better.

4. Come up with ideas for solutions and, by process of elimination, choose the best one.

Together, compile a list of realistic solutions that you will both feel positive about. Focus on the deeper emotional need behind the complaint. Think back to Mr. Thomas. His daughter's complaints of staff neglecting to feed her father stemmed out of a fear and guilt about his dying in an institutional setting. You could suggest she try to feed him with your supervision. This will both show her what you deal with daily and give her a sense of purpose and closeness in helping care for her father. Whatever the solution, make sure you come to it together and that you are both clear on your roles in it.

5. Agree to a time and place to try the solution and a time to look for a new solution, if necessary.

When a solution is agreed upon, determine together how you will note its progress. This means meetings in the future and specific goals to measure the effectiveness of the solution. For how long will you try it? What are some other possible solutions? With Mr. Thomas' daughter, you might have her come in 2-3 times a week, at different meal times, and monitor the progress. Remember, be specific about roles and trial lengths, so neither side can go back on their deal.

One of the most important steps of the process is setting a limited trial period on the solution. It needs a decent amount of time to see if it works, but not long enough that new problems develop. You and the family should have alternate solutions in mind ahead of time.

Making it through conflict and resolution with a family member can bring you closer together. It solves whatever the initial problem was, as well as giving them more faith in you as a caregiver.

Listen to this example, and then we'll try to solve it with our approach to resolving conflicts.

READ the following case study:

Mrs. Russell has been stuck in traffic on the way to the nursing home and is two hours late for a visit with her father. As she passes you in the hall, you ask, "How are you doing today, Mrs. Russell?" She snaps back at you, visibly angry.

"Not well, thank you. Frankly, I'm fed up with this place. I pay way too much money for inadequate service. I leave my father in this awful place, surrounded by filthy, drooling people. And what about the summer outfit I bought him? I've never even seen him wear it! You probably don't even know his name, always calling him "grandpa" and "dearie." I could do a much better job taking care of him myself, if I had the time."

Have members of your class act out this story, coming up with different scenarios and solutions.

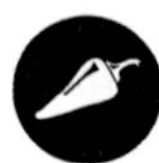

A Hot Idea

For a Class Exercise

Draft a complaint letter from a family member who lists numerous and specific complaints. Have the class members reply to the letter and decide what action should be taken to deal with each of the complaints. Have them either individually write out their responses or brainstorm out loud answers that you write on the board. Remind them to recall the module on communication as they do this exercise.

To conclude, SAY:

Think back to earlier in the class, when we listed positive and negative aspects of working with family. Think especially about the negative, challenging ones. How would we solve these now that we know more about resolving conflicts?

DISTRIBUTE Handout 9-3: QUIZ for Module 9.

Answers to the Module 9 Quiz:

1. True

2. True

3. True

4. False

5. False

6. True

7. True

8. True

9. False

10. True

The End...and a New Beginning

Congratulations! You and your class have now completed the entire career ladder program!

Before you celebrate, though, try to spend a few minutes reviewing the past nine modules with your class. What did they like most? Least? What would they like to learn more about? What was especially interesting or helpful?

Then ask the CNAs how they feel personally. Do they feel more professional? Proud of their position? Do they feel better equipped to deal with their jobs and other staff? Do they want to continue this learning? Do they feel they've changed over the course of the classes?

Once you've completed your discussion of the impact of the career ladder program, bring in your administrator to congratulate the class. Have him or her announce a time and place for their graduation ceremony. Make sure you urge your class to all come and to bring family and friends to witness their shining moment as they walk across the stage to receive their graduation certificate.

It's important to remember and stress a few important points when planning and implementing the graduation. One, the graduation acknowledges an important commitment by the CNA: an investment in herself and her career. Two, this is an achievement that benefits the residents, by ensuring that they are cared for by staff who possess the best skills available. The tips on the following page will give you some ideas for planning a graduation ceremony that celebrates this commitment and achievement in ways that are both fun and memorable.

Tips for Meaningful Graduation Celebrations

1. Invite elected officials and other dignitaries from your local community and have them participate in the graduation ceremony.
2. Work with these officials to create a proclamation declaring the day "Caregiver Day," and have it read aloud at the ceremony.
3. Provide graduates with attractive, framed certificates to honor their accomplishment.
4. Present each graduate with a pin to wear on his or her name-tag or collar.
5. Invite staff, residents, family, and friends to the ceremony.
6. Include special music.
7. Involve the residents from your facility in planning and conducting the graduation.
8. Provide refreshments, such as snacks, drinks, and cake.
9. Include a program for the event to hand out to attendees.
10. Invite local press to cover the event.
11. Consider photographing and videotaping the event.
12. Finally, use the event to show respect and thankfulness to the caregivers for their day-to-day commitment to excellent care and their own professional development.

Where Do We Go from Here?

Now that you have successfully completed your first career ladder program, you are on your way to building an effective continuous learning environment for the staff of your facility. Here are several steps that you can take to make ongoing learning opportunities a reality.

1. **Enlist recent career ladder graduates as co-creators of your learning community.** You have convinced your graduates that learning can be fun, valuable, and powerful. Now that they have completed the program, their ideas about their own training and learning needs can guide you as you envision and plan future training programs for the facility at large. You can think of their perspectives as a window into "the real world of the CNA." Think of ways to maintain an ongoing dialogue with them about continuous learning. You might want some of your graduates to serve on a facility committee to help plan your in-services or other training activities.

2. **Foster a career development vision for each CNA.** Look at this program as just the beginning of a path for the ongoing career development of your CNAs. Seriously consider developing a second tier or level of this program, so that any of your CNAs who graduate from your first level may have the opportunity to further develop their job skills and pursue areas of personal job interest and specialization. Again, enlist your graduates to assist in developing your program. What other topics do they need to know more about? What kinds of additional learning experiences do they need to support them in their jobs as professional, compassionate, and capable caregivers?

3. **Provide opportunities to participate in upcoming training events.** Think about ways to incorporate your graduates into future career ladder programs and other training events. They can provide valuable assistance, as helpers, with facilitation and planning. When you ask

your graduates whether or not they are interested in assisting you with upcoming training, make sure that they see their involvement as an opportunity to learn and develop their teaching skills, rather than as an obligation. Let them know that one of the best ways to continue learning is to teach.

Finally, think of these career ladder graduates as your most important asset. You have made an excellent initial investment in their professional development. Now you can protect that investment by partnering with them to build a work environment rich with continuous learning opportunities.

CNA
CAREER LADDER
MADE
EASY

Program Curriculum Handouts

HANDOUT 1-1

How to Wash Your Hands

The simplest and easiest way you can help prevent the spread of infection is by washing your hands. Here is a guide to when and how you should take this simple precaution.

WHEN TO WASH:

- Before and after you work with a resident.
- Before and after using medical/surgical or utility gloves.
- Before and after your shift.
- After touching dirty or contaminated clothing, sheets, or towels, which were in contact with body fluid.
- After touching anything where microorganisms are concentrated, like non-attached skin, any body fluid, wounds, and mucous membranes.
- After handling uncooked animal products, such as raw meat or fish.
- Before and after eating, handling food, or smoking.
- After coughing, sneezing, or blowing the nose.
- After using or assisting others with the bathroom, or after personal grooming.
- Before participating in a medical or surgical procedure.
- Whenever your hands look dirty.

WHAT YOU SHOULD USE TO WASH:

- When routinely washing for general patient/resident care, use ordinary soap, which includes lotion soap, liquid soap, powder soap, or bar soap. If you use a bar of soap, rinse it off first.

HANDOUT 1-1 *continued*

How to Wash Your Hands *continued*

WASHING YOUR HANDS:

- First moisten your hands with water, apply soap, and lather hands, wrists, and forearms.
- Rub your hands together for about 15 seconds (as long as it takes to sing two verses of Happy Birthday). Make sure you get in between the fingers, around and under nails and cuticles, and on the fronts and backs of your fingers. You must use friction when rubbing to remove organisms.
- Rinse your hands with warm running water.
- Dry your hands with a paper towel or air dryer. Turn on the air dryer with an elbow, never with your hands.
- Turn the faucet off with a paper towel to keep your hands from becoming contaminated again.
- Throw your paper towel in the trash to help others avoid contamination.

WHAT ABOUT HAND LOTIONS?

- You may use a lotion after washing your hands.
- Using a small, non-refillable container of lotion is preferable.
- If you will be using gloves later, do not use a petroleum-based product. These can decrease the effectiveness of the gloves, which protect your hands.
- Never use hand lotion if you will be participating in an invasive procedure.

REFERENCE:

Larson E. *APIC guideline for handwashing and hand antisepsis in health care settings.* AJIC 9/95; 23 (4); 251.

HANDOUT 1-2

Infection Control Terms

Biohazardous Material is anything infected with bodily fluids or certain poisonous medications.

Disinfection is a process that kills most bacteria, usually by means of washing with soap or treatment with chemicals.

Infection control is a process used to prevent the spread of micro-organisms that cause disease and infection among residents, employees, and visitors.

Nosocomial Infection is an infection acquired in a healthcare facility.

A **Pathogen** is an organism which causes disease. It can be a bacteria, fungus, or virus.

Sterilization is a process that kills all bacteria, usually through intense heat in a machine called an autoclave.

Universal Precautions are precautionary standards for providing care that contain and limit the spread of infection. They are comprised of specific steps to take when caring for all patients to avoid accidental contact with disease-carrying materials.

VRE/MRSA (Vancomycin Resistant Enterococcus/Methicillin resistant Staphylococcus aureus) are infections that resist most antibiotics.

HANDOUT 1-3

Types of Fire Extinguishers

FIRE EXTINGUISHERS ARE AS SIMPLE AS ABC...

There are two types of fire extinguishers and three types of fires. The key is knowing which extinguisher goes with which kind of fire.

TYPES OF EXTINGUISHERS:

Class A: A Class A extinguisher uses a stream of water.

Class ABC: A Class ABC extinguisher uses a white powder substance.

TYPES OF FIRES:

Class A: A Class A fire is one whose source is wood, paper, fabric, and any other substance that turns to ash. A Class A or Class ABC extinguisher should be used on this type of fire.

Class B: A Class B fire is one whose source is oil or grease. A Class ABC extinguisher should be used on this type of fire.

Class C: A Class C fire is an electrical fire. A Class ABC extinguisher should be used on this type of fire.

HANDOUT 1-4

Why Do Residents Fall?

A single disease, or a combination of many diseases, injuries, and disabilities can put a resident at a high risk of falling. Remember, a resident who has been bedridden or inactive because of an illness may be weaker and at a greater risk of falling. Some of the conditions that place an older person at greater risk are:

- Alzheimer's disease
- Arthritis
- Back problems
- Fever
- Impaired vision or hearing
- Inactivity, due to illness or injury
- Lung diseases, such as emphysema
- Parkinson's disease
- Stroke
- Drop in blood pressure
- Medications

HANDOUT 1-5

Environmental Risks

Here are some of the major environmental risks for falls:

- Highly polished linoleum or hardwood floors
- Worn carpeting and throw rugs
- Things placed haphazardly on the floor
- Poor lighting
- Wheelchairs
- Poorly maintained walkers or canes
- Poorly placed furniture
- Badly fitting shoes or clothing
- Power cords and thresholds in disrepair
- Water Spills
- Bedrails

HANDOUT 1-6

Back Injury: The Top Causes

Poor planning. Failing to test or size up a load, check the travel path, or clear an area for the object to be placed on often leads to additional stress on the back.

Handling the load from far away. The stress on the body increases seven to ten times when a load is at arms length, compared to lifting something close to the body.

Twisting and bending at the same time. Not pivoting the feet or squatting to lift causes maximum stress on the lower back.

Lifting with the back bent forward and the legs straight. This places too much stress on the support structures of the lower back.

Using fast jerking motions. Lifting objects which are hard to grip, working in an area with slipping and tripping hazards, or trying to work too fast can prevent smooth, safe technique.

Lack of assistive devices. A piece of equipment is often required to move objects safely and without it, the movement is unsafe. Employees should know if they are available and, more importantly, how to use them.

Poor communication. When two people are lifting together, they should coordinate their movement. Misunderstanding instructions can also result in unnecessary risk.

Rushing. Not asking for help because you're in a hurry puts you at a higher risk for back injury.

THINK — AND THEN LIFT!

HANDOUT 1-7

Five Steps to a Safe Transfer

1. **Greet the resident.** Tell them why you are there. If it is the first time you will perform this move, give a brief explanation of it. Ask them how much assistance will they require? Do they have an accurate sense of their own abilities? Remember, encourage their independence as much as possible. Pay attention to their feelings. If they don't feel secure and comfortable, try to put them at ease. A transfer is not something you do to the resident, or even for the resident, but **with** the resident.

2. **Plan the move.** First, evaluate what you will need. Another person? A piece of equipment? Never use time-saving as a reason to do a difficult lift alone. Place the bed, chair, wheelchair, commode, or stretcher in the correct position. Make sure the wheelchair is locked. Map out where you will stand, where you will grasp the resident, and how you will move your feet once the transfer is underway. Always visualize the transfer before you carry it out to work out all your moves.

3. **Communicate throughout the transfer.** Keeping clear communication will reduce the chance for injury. Ask the resident if they are prepared for the move, if they are comfortable during the move, and whether they are ready for the next step of the move. Tell them what you're doing before and while you do it. Keep a running conversation with any assisting co-worker. Confer about each step and let them know how they can best help you.

4. **Observe the resident for any change** in her abilities, and also for any signs of pain. Noting these changes will let you know if you have to alter your transferring technique. It will also provide you with information for the larger picture. Note any changes in behavior, also. These could be important in later planning for that resident.

5. **Document the transfer** including what equipment was used, and how many staff were involved. This documentation is necessary for your supervisor to fill out the MDS form accurately.

HANDOUT 1-8

Know Your Transfer Equipment

Make sure you know when and how to use this equipment:

Use a **drawsheet** to transfer a resident who must remain lying down. You will need a co-worker to use this tool. Never use a drawsheet to transfer a resident with a back injury or the possibility of one.

Use a **hydraulic lift** with heavier residents, residents who are not weight-bearing, or when other staff are not available for assistance. The wheels on a hydraulic lift are only for moving it into position — never use the hydraulic lift to transport a resident over any distance.

A **slide board** is a smooth plank of wood (or other strong material) that is placed across two surfaces at equal height. Then the resident is assisted in sliding along the board from one surface to another; for example, from bed to wheelchair.

Place a **transfer** or **gait belt** around the resident's waist to give you something secure to grip during a transfer. This can be helpful when transferring a resident with a poor sense of balance.

Use a **transfer board,** a full-length board, to transfer a resident who must remain lying down with his back perfectly straight. Generally, you use this to move residents with spinal or back injuries.

A **trapeze bar** is simply a bar that hangs from a frame over the resident's bed. Residents can use it to raise and exercise their upper body from the bed.

HANDOUT 1-9

The Pivot Transfer

Pivot transfers are the most common kind of transfer used in a nursing facility. It allows you to move a disabled resident from bed to chair/wheelchair/commode and back again by yourself. This example will use a bed to wheelchair pivot transfer:

1. Encourage the resident to help.
2. Position the wheelchair at a right angle and as close as possible to the bed on the resident's strong side. Raise the footrests, and make sure the wheels are locked.
3. Adjust the resident's bed to the lowest position that is level with the wheelchair and raise the head of the bed to help them into a sitting position. Lower bed rail if necessary.
4. Help the resident into a sitting position with their feet on the floor.
5. Stand knee to knee in front of the resident and put your arms under their arms, or grasp the transfer belt.
6. Use your knees to support the resident as you help them stand.
7. Pivot in the direction of the wheelchair, slowly, being careful to shift the position of your feet several times. Do not twist your body at the hips.
8. Position the resident and lower them into the wheelchair. Place the resident's feet on the footrests, and make sure they are comfortable.

HANDOUT 1-10

QUIZ for Module 1

1. The best way to move a resident from their wheelchair to their bed is bend, lift, and twist at the hips. ❑ True ❑ False

2. Blood, feces, and urine should always be assumed infectious.
❑ True ❑ False

3. A transfer is only complete when the resident is comfortable in their destination.
❑ True ❑ False

4. Falls can not be caused by loose clothing.
❑ True ❑ False

5. The majority of resident falls take place in the dining room.
❑ True ❑ False

6. Infection is one of the leading causes of death among the aged.
❑ True ❑ False

7. Only a sick person can carry a harmful pathogen.
❑ True ❑ False

8. Back injuries are usually caused by a single occurrence.
❑ True ❑ False

9. A nosocomial infection is an infection of the nasal passages.
❑ True ❑ False

10. Looking on a resident's floor for trouble can prevent a fall.
❑ True ❑ False

HANDOUT 2-1

The Center of the Team

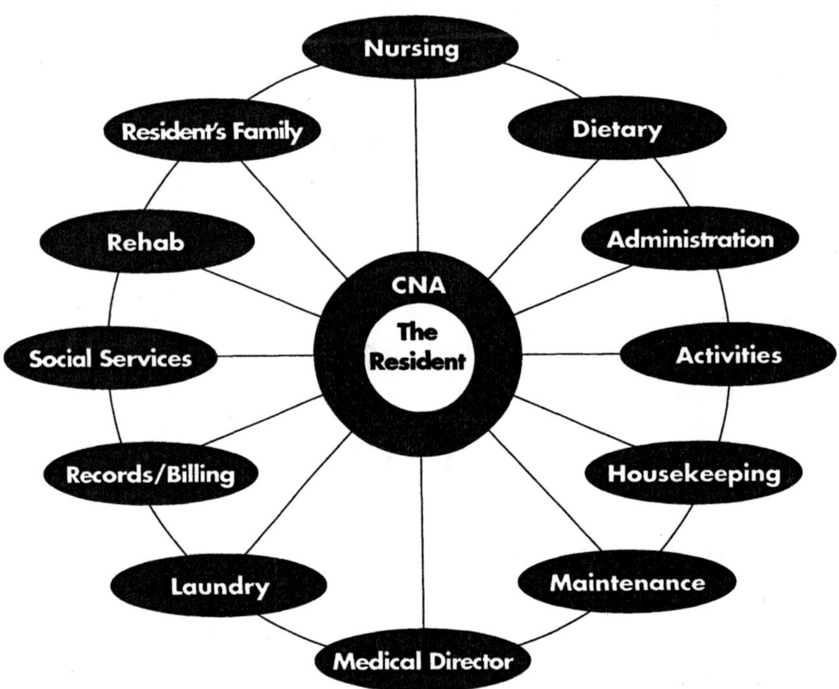

HANDOUT 2-2

The Five Functions of a Team

1. Setting goals

Teams have to be able to identify priorities and determine the amount of time needed to complete these tasks. In a long term care facility, a team must identify their specific tasks, determine which of the tasks is a priority, and approximate the time necessary to complete them.

2. Distributing assignments

Once the tasks are identified and prioritized, the team must decide — based on each person's skills, competence, and team acceptance — who will accomplish those tasks. Understanding the nature of roles, assessing the needs of the facility and its residents, and determining who is going to perform those tasks require substantial team effort.

3. Establishing standard procedures

Any attempted task — from lifting a resident to recording ADLs — requires a process. Teams develop ways to make decisions, resolve conflicts, assign leadership, communicate, and establish team norms.

4. Maintaining good relationships

Trust, support, respect, and comfort among all team members are essential for a team's success. The level of trust that exists among team members determines the levels of respect and comfort each team member will feel for other members of the team. Trust and support build as each member understands the larger vision of the organization.

5. Dealing with conflicts

Conflict arises when one team member's goals do not match the goals of the team. In order for the team to operate effectively and successfully carry out its tasks, the individual's and team's objectives must be compatible.

HANDOUT 2-3

Think SMART

When setting your team's goal, think SMART:

S — **Specific**
Be as clear and specific as you can about the goal.

M — **Measurable**
There should be a way to tell whether or not you have reached the goal.

A — **Attainable**
Set high goals but not too high; make sure it is a goal you can reach.

R — **Realistic**
The goal should take into account your resources, and the strengths and weaknesses of the team.

T — **Timely**
The goal should be formed so that it can be accomplished within several months, and in no longer than a year.

HANDOUT 2-4

Mrs. Jones

Pamela Jones is 82 years old and just entered Fresh Pond Nursing Home two weeks ago. For the last three years since her husband died, she lived with her daughter. Her daughter had a harder and harder time caring for her mom at home because Mrs. Jones was getting so confrontational, and then so depressed. So, her daughter decided it was best that her mother go live at Fresh Pond, most likely as a permanent residence.

In the past, Mrs. Jones has been hospitalized because she would forget to take her medication, or she would take too much. She has a history of diabetes, which is controlled by adherence to a strict diet, and congestive heart disease, for which her physician has prescribed Lanoxin and Lasix. Her doctor says her forgetfulness could be due to the onset of AD-type dementia. Recently, her doctors have determined that Mrs. Jones has developed osteoarthritis.

After meeting with Mrs. Jones and her daughter, the interdisciplinary team learned some important things, such as Mrs. Jones was married for fifty years and had been a stay home mother her entire married life; they had four children; her husband had worked as a shoe salesman; and they had never left the town where they had grown up, met, and got married. Mrs. Jones is a member of St. John's Episcopal Church, where she has been an active volunteer for the past 15 years, and she volunteered at her local library for almost thirty years. She has many other interests, such as: knitting, gardening, exploring tag sales, reading all kinds of books, and has a big collection of her grandchildren's drawings and letters.

Those at the facility feel that Mrs. Jones is adjusting well to the facility, though her memory has been slowly deteriorating. This is most troubling, because she likes to keep in touch with her children and grandchildren, and is forgetting to do so. Because of arthritis, she has a hard time writing, closing envelopes, and applying stamps. Recently she confessed to her daughter that she feared losing touch with, or even worse, forgetting about her family. This thought causes her such dejection that she is starting to lose hope and has said, "soon, I won't even know myself anymore."

HANDOUT 2-5

A Sample Care Plan

Use this basic form in conjunction with Handout 2-4 to develop a sample care plan.

RESIDENT: Pamela Jones		
PROBLEM	GOAL	INTERVENTION

HANDOUT 2-6

QUIZ for Module 2

1. A good team is made of people all exactly like you.
   ❑ True ❑ False

2. Being on a team makes the work more fun.
   ❑ True ❑ False

3. As a CNA, you are only a member of the clinical team.
   ❑ True ❑ False

4. Some jobs are just too large or complex for an individual.
   ❑ True ❑ False

5. One of the functions of a team is to deal with conflicts.
   ❑ True ❑ False

6. A team is a group of people with a variety of different skills, talents, and experiences working toward a shared goal. ❑ True ❑ False

7. Teamwork is okay, but it isn't essential to a resident's care.
   ❑ True ❑ False

8. A team has to prioritize and determine the amount of time required to complete certain tasks.
   ❑ True ❑ False

9. The best teams just appear magically.
   ❑ True ❑ False

10. Along with RNs, LPNs, various therapists, and your facility's Medical Director, you are a member of the clinical team. ❑ True ❑ False

HANDOUT 2-7

Tips for Panelists

THANK YOU for being a part of our CNA Career Ladder program.

You will serve on a panel of representatives from various departments throughout the facility. After brief presentations, there will be questions and a class discussion. Your visit to the class will help to demonstrate the spirit of teamwork that we want to foster in our facility and which is the theme of the module your presentation will be part of.

The panel will meet on _______ (date), at _______ o'clock, in _______ (room). Please don't be late.

Please arrange about 3-5 minutes worth of comments. Here are some areas you should address:

- The function of your department.
- Who the people are in it.
- What kind of training they have.
- How you and your department can work together with CNAs in resident care.
- Can the nursing assistants help you and your department operate better?
- Who in your department would a nursing assistant contact with a question or problem?

Thanks again for your time and effort. See you on the _____th.

Sincerely,

HANDOUT 3-1

The Physical Changes of Aging

- Slower metabolism
- Dehydration
- Constipation
- Reduced energy level
- Weight change
- Bone density loss
- Height loss
- Hair changes: graying, thinning, balding
- Physical discomfort
- Fatigue
- Stooped posture
- Appetite loss
- Sensory perception loss
- Changing sleep patterns
- Skin tears more common

HANDOUT 3-2

Diabetic Warning Signs

WARNING SIGNS OF

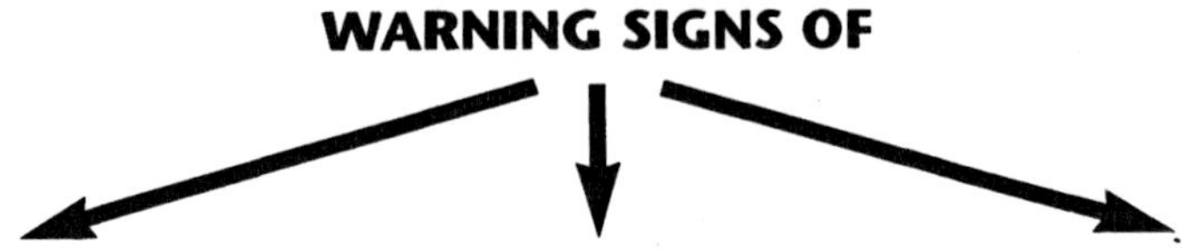

HIGH BLOOD SUGAR

- Weakness/fatigue
- Increased appetite or thirst
- Frequent urination
- Blurred vision
- Slow healing of wounds or sores
- Dry, itchy skin
- Confusion
- Headache

LOW BLOOD SUGAR

- Shakiness, trembling
- Sweatiness
- Anxiety, irritability
- Impaired vision
- Disorientation
- Headache

DEHYDRATION

- Dry mouth
- Thirst
- Sunken eyes
- Dark, strong-smelling urine
- Speech difficulty/verbal confusion
- Constipation
- Headache

HANDOUT 3-3

Osteoarthritis

CAUSES

- Wear and tear on the joint
- Repeated injury or infection of the joint
- Genetic; it runs in the family

SYMPTOMS

- Joint pain, especially after exercise
- Joint stiffness, especially after inactivity
- Aching, commonly during weather changes
- Grating, due to increased roughness of bones
- Fluid accumulation; fluid collects and needs draining
- Limitation of movement
- Joint deformity, redness, or enlargement
- Destruction of joint

HANDOUT 3-4

Hip Surgery Precautions

A resident who has just undergone hip surgery is in a very delicate condition. Here are some precautions you can take with them:

- **Prevent** the hip from moving past **90** degrees.
- Frequently change their position to improve circulation, prevent pressure ulcers, and give relief to muscles and bones.
- Fully support the operated area during moves.
- Rotate them in one movement, from back to side and side to back.
- Observe weight-bearing instructions.
- Use an abductor pillow or wedge to maintain alignment. (Demonstrate to the class.)
- Do not let them bend from the waist or cross legs.
- Make sure their back is straight when they rise.

HANDOUT 3-5

Possible Signs of Stroke

If you observe one or more of these signs of a stroke in a resident, REPORT YOUR OBSERVATION IMMEDIATELY:

- **Sudden numbness or weakness** of face, arm or leg, especially on one side of the body.
- **Sudden confusion,** trouble speaking or understanding.
- **Sudden trouble seeing** in one or both eyes.
- **Sudden trouble walking,** dizziness, loss of balance or coordination.
- **Sudden severe headache** with no known cause.

HANDOUT 3-6

Care for Stroke Patients

You can help care for your residents who have suffered a stroke by:

- Encouraging exercise of joints to prevent atrophy and contractures.
- Re-positioning them to avoid bed sores.
- Giving them good skin care.
- Taking safety measures, like using bed rails and walkers.
- Allowing time for them to communicate and using communication aids when necessary.
- Providing progressive self-feeding.
- Encouraging participation, promoting independence.

They might also receive other treatments, like:

- Speech therapy.
- ADL re-training.
- Restorative therapy.

HANDOUT 3-7

QUIZ for Module 3

1. Diabetes is an illness that affects approximately one-fifth of all people over 65.
   ❑ True ❑ False

2. A stroke occurs when blood circulation to the brain fails.
   ❑ True ❑ False

3. Usually osteoarthritis is found throughout the body.
   ❑ True ❑ False

4. There are two types of diabetes: Type I and Type II.
   ❑ True ❑ False

5. As a CNA, your job is to diagnose illness.
   ❑ True ❑ False

6. Typical symptoms of rheumatoid arthritis include: weight gain and low body temperature.
   ❑ True ❑ False

7. The type of arthritis that most often afflicts the elderly is osteoarthritis.
   ❑ True ❑ False

8. Several of the typical changes of normal aging include appetite loss and reduced energy level.
   ❑ True ❑ False

9. Diabetes is sometimes known as "no blood sugar."
   ❑ True ❑ False

10. The three stages in the treatment of a stroke victim are flaccid, spastic, and recovery.
    ❑ True ❑ False

HANDOUT 4-1

Test Your Communication Skills

How do your communication skills add up?
Answer yes or no to these statements and see.

1. I communicate my expectations clearly. ❑ Yes ❑ No

2. My body language gives the same message that my voice gives. ❑ Yes ❑ No

3. I summarize the other person's problem to show them I am listening.
   ❑ Yes ❑ No

4. I am sincere when speaking with residents. ❑ Yes ❑ No

5. I always answer family member's questions as if they had just asked them for the first time. ❑ Yes ❑ No

6. I maintain eye contact while talking to others. ❑ Yes ❑ No

7. I give non-verbal cues, like nodding, to show someone I understand what they are saying. ❑ Yes ❑ No

8. I interrupt others when they are speaking. ❑ Yes ❑ No

HANDOUT 4-2

Communication Roadblocks

Labeling the person in a generalizing or stereotypical way.
("He's such a Southerner, so slow and lazy.")

Threatening the other person.
("Take care of that mess or I'll tell your supervisor!")

Offering unsolicited advice.
("You definitely need to tell that resident's mother how you're feeling.")

Using morals as a defense.
("If her daughter really loved her mother, she wouldn't have put her here.")

Ordering the person around.
("Go attend to Mrs. Welsh right now!")

Trying to redirect or ignore someone's problem.
("Why don't you go talk to Nancy, I'm too busy.")

Blaming the other person.
("Your father's behavior is totally your fault.")

Using "always" and "never."
("Why do you always come in late?" "You never help at mealtime.")

Calling the person names.
("Polly is such an airhead.")

HANDOUT 4-3

Follow the Yellow Brick Road

Follow every direction below, step by step.

1. Read every step below before you proceed with the following directions.
2. Write down the name of your instructor at the top left corner of this page.
3. Multiply 56 by 73.
4. Add 1290 to this number.
5. Draw smiley faces on every zero of the answer to Step 4.
6. Write the name of your favorite food in the lower left corner.
7. Draw a big circle on the back of the page.
8. Draw a smaller circle inside the circle from Step 7.
9. Stick out your tongue at the person sitting to your right.
10. Divide the result of Step 4 by 39.
11. Write your mother's first name on the top right hand corner.
12. Add 45935 to the result of Step 10
13. Draw a box around the answer to Step 12.
14. Clap your hands 3 times.
15. Draw a picture of face saying "yum" next to your answer from Step 6.
16. Color in all the O's on the page.
17. If you have done everything correctly to this point, "moo" out loud.
18. Cross out Step 8.
19. Sign your name along the side of the page.
20. Do not do anything after Step 1.

HANDOUT 4-4

Three Types of Feedback

1. EMOTION-BASED FEEDBACK

Let the person know you understand how they are feeling. For example, "You're stressed out because you just sat in traffic for an hour. I know how frustrating that can be."

2. FACT-BASED FEEDBACK

Recount what you think is being said in a factual way. For example, "You were late for your shift because there was a traffic jam on the turnpike."

3. SOLUTION-BASED FEEDBACK

Try to come up with a solution to that person's problem. For example, "Maybe you should try taking the bus to work. It's much quicker and you wouldn't have to worry about parking."

HANDOUT 4-5

"I-Messages"

When __________________________ happens,

I feel ___________________________

because ________________________.

I would like _____________________ to happen.

HANDOUT 4-6

Tony and Mrs. Li

Tony is a young, burly Italian CNA from New York City with a voice that booms through the facility. He loves greeting the residents, and is about to meet Mrs. Li for the first time. Mrs. Li is originally from Japan.

He enters the room, saying "I hear there's a lovely new lady here. I've just got to meet her." With a huge grin and his hand out for a handshake, he approaches her, "Mrs. Li! Glad to meet you. I'm Tony. Can I call you Joan? I think we're gonna get along wonderfully."

Mrs. Li does not move. She doesn't say a word or even look in Tony's direction. She holds her hands tightly in her lap. Tony continues, "Hey Joan, don't be shy. Let's be friends," and puts out his hand again. Mrs. Li turns her head away from him.

Tony is confused and a little hurt. His openness usually works with the residents and he can't understand why Mrs. Li won't respond to him.

What could be the problem here? Could there be a conflict of cultures?

HANDOUT 4-7

Cultural Communication Tips

1. Try to make friends with people of other cultural groups.

2. Learn about other people's customs, holidays, and religious practices. Ask them about these things and share some of your own with them.

3. Think about your own feelings towards another cultural group. Do you have any prejudices or stereotypes? Where do these feelings come from?

4. Don't allow the people around you to use cultural stereotypes. Think of how you would feel if someone mindlessly insulted your background.

5. Try to learn some important words from another language. Use them when around people that speak that language.

6. Observe how people within a culture interact with one another. How do people in your culture interact with each other? (For instance, do you kiss on both cheeks when you greet someone or do you formally bow?) How are the two cultures different?

HANDOUT 4-8

Betty and Maureen

Betty and Maureen have worked together as CNAs for five years. During the last week, Betty has been back late from her break three times, causing frustration for Maureen and some of the other CNAs who have had to pick up her responsibilities. Maureen confronts Betty on the third day and says:

"Do you ever think about anyone but yourself? We all have to cover for you every time. And then you saunter in 15 minutes late like nothing happened!"

HANDOUT 4-9

QUIZ for Module 4

1. Fact-based feedback is useful, because it clarifies that you've understood the conversation. ❑ True ❑ False

2. When it comes to emotional issues, feedback is useless. ❑ True ❑ False

3. Body language can be as important a communication tool as language.
❑ True ❑ False

4. Making fun of people from different cultures makes everyone feel comfortable.
❑ True ❑ False

5. Listening well and speaking calmly are especially difficult under stress.
❑ True ❑ False

6. While listening to someone talk, you should be planning your response.
❑ True ❑ False

7. The majority of conflicts arise from misunderstandings.
❑ True ❑ False

8. Calling people names is an effective communication tool. ❑ True ❑ False

9. The most important part of "active listening" is to stay calm and evaluate the speaker's emotional state. ❑ True ❑ False

10. Culture can be defined completely by food, music, and clothing.
❑ True ❑ False

HANDOUT 5-1

The Pyramid of Food

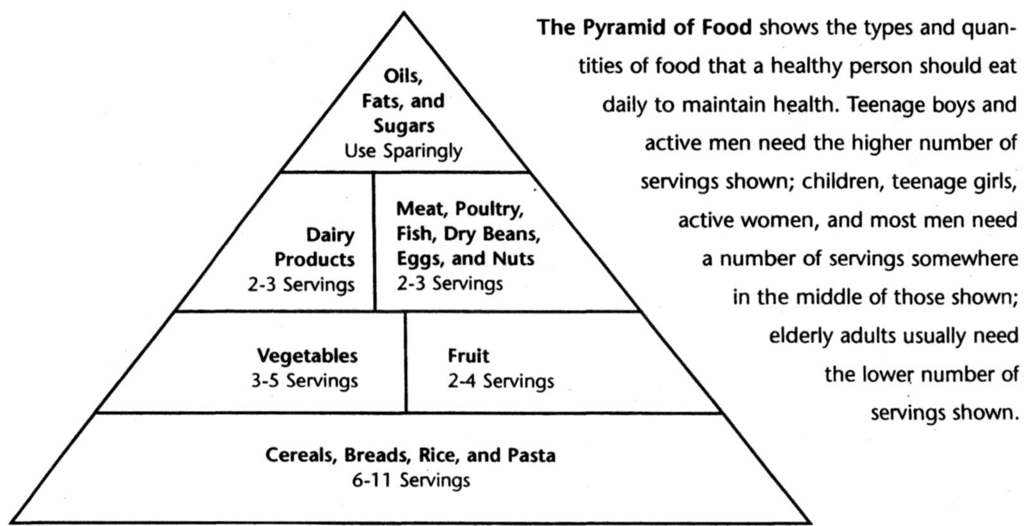

The Pyramid of Food shows the types and quantities of food that a healthy person should eat daily to maintain health. Teenage boys and active men need the higher number of servings shown; children, teenage girls, active women, and most men need a number of servings somewhere in the middle of those shown; elderly adults usually need the lower number of servings shown.

A Single Serving of Each Group Equals...

Cereals, Breads, Rice, and Pasta
- 1 slice of bread
- 1 cup of cooked pasta or rice
- 1 cup of hot cereal
- 1 ounce of cold cereal

Fruits
- 1 piece of fruit or wedge of melon
- 1 cup of fruit juice
- 1 cup of canned fruit

Oils, Fats, and Sugars
- Limit calories from these, especially if weight loss is needed

Vegetables
- 1 cup, chopped vegetables
- 1 cup of leafy raw vegetables

Dairy Products
- 1 cup of milk or yogurt
- 1 to 2 ounces of cheese

Meat, Poultry, Fish, Legumes, Eggs, and Nuts
- 2 to 3 ounces of cooked lean meat, poultry, or fish
- 1 cup of cooked beans, or 1 egg, or 2 tablespoons of peanut butter equal 1 ounce of lean meat (approx. 2 of a serving).

HANDOUT 5-2

Symptoms of Nutritional Disease

1. **Loss of:**
    - appetite
    - hair
    - taste or smell
    - balance
    - weight (or gain in weight)
    - breath, upon exertion or at rest
    - memory

2. **Pain, discomfort, or soreness:**
    - when eating or swallowing
    - in lips, tongue, or throat
    - in stomach, causing vomiting

3. **Changes in:**
    - bowel habits (diarrhea, constipation, bloody, bulky, or foul-smelling stools)
    - light sensitivity
    - healing times of wounds, sores, and ulcers
    - skin color

4. **Depression**

5. **Bruising**

HANDOUT 5-3

The DETERMINE List

D

DISEASE
Any disease, illness, or ongoing condition which changes the way a resident eats, or makes it hard for a resident to eat, puts him or her at nutritional risk. Confusion or memory loss can make it hard to remember what, when, or if one has eaten. Feeling sad or depressed can cause big changes in appetite, digestion, energy level, weight, and well-being.

E

EATING POORLY
Eating too little and eating too much both lead to poor health. Eating the same foods day after day or not eating fruit, vegetables, and milk products daily will also cause poor nutritional health. Many health problems become worse when people drink more than one or two alcoholic beverages per day.

T

TOOTH LOSS/MOUTH PAIN
A healthy mouth, teeth, and gums are needed to eat. Missing, loose or rotten teeth or dentures that don't fit well or cause mouth sores make it hard to eat.

E

ECONOMIC HARDSHIP
Many older Americans have low incomes. It is very hard to get the food needed to stay healthy with less than $25-30 per week.

R

REDUCED SOCIAL CONTACT
Being with other people has a positive effect on eating habits because social activity improves morale and well-being.

M

MULTIPLE MEDICINES
Many older Americans must take medicines for health problems. Almost half of older Americans take multiple medicines daily. Growing old may change the way we respond to drugs. The more medicines an elderly person takes, the greater the chance for side effects such as increased or decreased appetite, change in taste, constipation, weakness, drowsiness, diarrhea, or nausea. Vitamins or minerals when taken in large doses act like drugs and can cause harm.

I

INVOLUNTARY WEIGHT LOSS/GAIN
Losing or gaining a lot of weight when a resident is not trying to do so is an important warning signal that must not be ignored. Being overweight or underweight also increases a resident's chance of poor health.

N

NEEDS ASSISTANCE IN SELF-CARE
People who require more assistance are likely to have eating problems.

E

ELDER YEARS ABOVE AGE 80
Most older people lead full and productive lives. But as age increases, risk of frailty and health problems increase. Regularly checking the nutritional status of nursing home residents over the age of 80 makes sense.

(From the Report of Nutrition Screening 1: Toward a Common View, Executive Summary, Washington, D.C., The Nutrition Screening Initiative.)

HANDOUT 5-4

Loss of Appetite

For residents of nursing homes, appetite loss can happen for many reasons, such as:

- medications that have side-effects like nausea, dry mouth, and decreased ability to taste and smell
- digestive problems, including heartburn, diarrhea, and constipation
- chronic pain
- chronic disease or disability, such as arthritis, diabetes, dementia, and depression
- dental or denture problems
- social anxiety
- poor eating environment, such as a noisy, stressful dining room
- unappetizing or cold food

HANDOUT 5-5

Calories

Calories come from carbohydrates, proteins, and fats. Most foods contain calories from more than a single source.

1 gram of carbohydrate = 4 calories

1 gram of protein = 4 calories

1 gram of fat = 9 calories

For people between the ages of 51 and 75, caloric needs reduce by ten percent. After 75, these needs decrease another ten to fifteen percent, depending on their activity levels.

As a person ages, their energy needs decrease, because their lean body mass and level of activity decreases. Caloric needs depend on one's activity level as well as their body composition, so a bedridden resident requires less calories than an active one.

Through exercise, older people keep their lean body mass, though it can still decrease even in those people who exercise often. A person can eat more without gaining weight, the more lean body mass they have. The higher their lean body mass, the more likely they will get enough nutrients.

REMEMBER:
Older adults may need less calories, but they have a greater need for certain nutrients. These nutrients must be obtained with a lower intake of food, as older adults tend to eat less than younger ones. Discourage foods with little nutritional value, like sugar and alcohol. Encourage nutrient-rich food, like vegetables, fruit, low fat milk and dairy, lean meat, fish, whole grains, and poultry.

HANDOUT 5-6

Mr. Parks

Mr. Parks has what he likes to call a "healthy appetite." He will eat anything. His "ideal breakfast" would be steak and eggs, toast smothered in butter, homefries, maybe even a side of bacon. And coffee, with lots of cream and extra sugar. He is happy to lend a helping hand, or mouth, in the dining room to residents with lesser appetites.

When it's not mealtime, Mr. Parks stays in his room, taking numerous naps and snapping at staff and other residents who try to talk to him. He demands sweets from the staff and is enraged when he is denied. Sometimes, he even yells and threatens the CNAs.

One CNA recently reported that she thinks Mr. Parks could be suffering from AD-type dementia. His anger and threats are increasing lately, and he often appears to not remember them afterwards.

HANDOUT 5-7

Mealtime Checklist

- Wash resident's hands prior to mealtime.
- Always promote a friendly environment at mealtime.
- Make sure the resident's clothing is protected.
- Know and monitor your resident's food preferences.
- Offer a substitute if the resident declines a meal.
- Give the name of each food and beverage that you serve.
- For residents with vision problems, give the food locations on their plate.
- Make sure that cold foods are cold and hot foods are hot.
- Warn the resident if foods and liquids are hot.
- Ask if the resident is full at the end of the meal.
- Help with oral care after the meal.
- Toilet the resident before a mealtime.
- Help clean the resident after the meal, with a cloth or change of clothes.

HANDOUT 5-8

QUIZ for Module 5

1. Fruit that is canned in syrup is especially nutritious.
   ❑ True ❑ False

2. Vegetables such as spinach, broccoli, cauliflower, and kale are rich in cancer-blocking chemicals. ❑ True ❑ False

3. The majority of older adults get all the calcium they need.
   ❑ True ❑ False

4. Caffeinated and alcoholic beverages can act as diuretics.
   ❑ True ❑ False

5. The right amounts of fruits, vegetables, dairy, fiber, protein, and water makes up a healthy diet. ❑ True ❑ False

6. Problems that can be traced to poor nutrition require medication to improve.
   ❑ True ❑ False

7. Without enough water, blood pressure can drop dangerously low.
   ❑ True ❑ False

8. As a rule, making sure social atmosphere, the physical environment, and the food are all appealing will contribute to nutritional well-being.
   ❑ True ❑ False

9. If a person has lost their appetite, there's no way you can help them.
   ❑ True ❑ False

10. Malnutrition is strictly the result of a diet too low in calories.
    ❑ True ❑ False

HANDOUT 6-1

Religious Holidays

Different religions observe their holy days at different times, as many religions have different calendars than the one we're used to. By knowing when and how their religious days are celebrated, you can show residents you are interested in their spirituality. Here are names and short descriptions of some of the major holidays:

- **Chinese New Year:** a time of celebration and gift giving during the new moon nearest to the fifteenth degree of Aquarius.
- **Christmas:** December 25th, the celebration of the birth of Christ and a time for family and gift giving.
- **Feast of Ridván:** the observance of the declaration of prophethood by Bahá'u'lláh, prophet-founder of the Bahá'í Faith, between April 21 and May 2.
- **Hanukkah:** the Jewish Feast of Dedication, which is observed for eight days, in commemoration of the rededication of the Jerusalem Temple in 164 B.C., a time of lighting candles, reciting benedictions, and giving gifts.
- **Kwanzaa:** the African-American celebration for giving thanks, between December 26th and January 1st; the first day of Kwanzaa is called Umoja (unity); the holiday has its origins as an African harvest celebration.
- **Lent:** the season leading up to the Christian celebration of Easter.
- **Native American feast days:** these special days vary from tribe to tribe, and are usually days of prayers, dancing, and opening up of homes for guests, meals, and celebration.
- **Ramadan:** the ninth month of the Muslim calendar, in which believers fast daily from dawn to sunset.
- **Yom Kippur:** the most solemn day of the Jewish calendar, also called the Day of Atonement, a day of prayer and fasting, occurring in the seventh month of the Jewish calendar.

HANDOUT 6-2

When a Resident is Dying

A dying resident has many particular needs that set them apart from other residents. They include:

- talking
- feeling like a "normal" person until the end
- perceiving meaning in death
- sharing and coming to terms with their inescapable future
- being with a caring person as they die
- freedom from pain as much as possible
- the opportunity to voice their fears
- someone to listen with compassion and understanding
- visit by clergyman

HANDOUT 6-3

The Five Stages of Dying

Dr. Kubler-Ross's five stages of dying:

STAGE 1: DENIAL

In this stage, the resident will not accept their coming death. Do not argue with them or try to correct their attitude. Just listen to their feelings and fears as they try to come to terms with their situation.

STAGE 2: ANGER

When the person accepts that they are dying, they often become angry at their fate. A resident who was once gentle and quiet could become confrontational and abusive in this period. They may express anger at you, their family, even God. They may irrationally blame or attack you, but you need to see this anger for what it really is: They are keeping death and the unknown at bay with a mask of anger.

STAGE 3: BARGAINING

As they face the inevitability of death, some people will start bargaining for continued life. They may offer to stop doing one thing or start another in exchange for more time. Often this is done silently. If a resident does it aloud and tries to involve you, be understanding and patient. Here is an example:

> Dying patient: *I'll stop lying and being such a mean person, if I could just live to see my granddaughter graduate from college.*
>
> Your response: *I see how strongly you feel about this graduation. Would you like to tell me why it's so important to you. I'd be interested in hearing about it.*

HANDOUT 6-3 *continued*

The Five Stages of Dying *continued*

STAGE 4: DEPRESSION

In this stage, after the person has realized they cannot bargain their way out of or avoid dying, they will often become depressed. They may refuse food, water, and medication. They may avoid interaction with other people or simply shut down mentally. Trying to cheer them up is not a good idea.They begin to acknowledge that their feelings are justified and appropriate for their situation. They may eventually want someone to talk to about their situation, and you should be a willing listener.

STAGE 5: ACCEPTANCE

After the emotional roller-coaster of the last four stages, most people emerge to accept their situation. During this stage, the resident will probably want to be left alone or with a small group of family and friends as they await death. The best thing for you to do, as a CNA, is to be there when you are needed. Do not force the resident into conversation or unnecessary interaction. Be intuitive, learn to anticipate the needs of your resident and their family. Help them remain as comfortable as possible in their final days, quietly and with care.

HANDOUT 6-4

Your Beliefs

What are your beliefs regarding dying and death?

1. If you were told you had three months to live, what would you do with your time?

2. What defines a "good death" for you?

3. If you were dying, what would your needs be from family and friends?

4. What religious beliefs do you have about death and dying?

5. If someone you love was dying, who would you turn to for strength and comfort?

6. If you were asked to assist a dying resident, which of your values and beliefs about death and dying would be hardest to put aside?

HANDOUT 6-5

The Stages of Grief

There are several common experiences and stages that grieving people share:

1. **Disbelief and shock.**

   Initial reactions to a loved one's death are usually disbelief and shock. At first, they may feel numb and even emotionless.

2. **Yearning.**

   When the disbelief fades, yearning for the lost loved one often sets in. They intensely miss the person, even to the point of hearing their voice or seeing an illusion of them. At this point, they may also feel guilty and irritable.

3. **Depression.**

   A period of depression and emotional instability usually follows.

4. **Recovery.**

   In the end, a period of recovery should ensue. They become able to think of themselves without that person and begin to fill in the spaces that this death has created in their life.

HANDOUT 6-6

QUIZ for Module 6

1. Yom Kippur can also be called the Day of Atonement.
   ❑ True ❑ False

2. If a favorite resident dies, you should just ignore it and go about your day.
   ❑ True ❑ False

3. Grief is the way we respond to the loss of a loved one, as well as the way we recover from that loss. ❑ True ❑ False

4. You should leave dying residents alone. ❑ True ❑ False

5. A dying person must go through Kubler-Ross's five stages in the correct order.
   ❑ True ❑ False

6. You should not concern yourself with residents' religious beliefs.
   ❑ True ❑ False

7. Part of your role as a CNA is seeing that residents' spiritual needs are met.
   ❑ True ❑ False

8. As they experience many losses later in life, the elderly often turn to their spirituality for comfort and strength. ❑ True ❑ False

9. Kwanzaa happens around the same time as Christmas.
   ❑ True ❑ False

10. One's spiritual beliefs must be expressed through religious ritual.
    ❑ True ❑ False

HANDOUT 7-1

The New Resident

1. ***Review the list below and put a check next to all the things you enjoy about your independence.***

__ Going to sleep and waking on your own schedule.

__ Talking privately on the phone.

__ Deciding what and when you want to eat.

__ Having a glass of wine with dinner.

__ Visiting with friends.

__ Keeping house plants.

__ Sleeping in a king-size bed.

__ Having a pet.

__ Taking a walk around the block.

__ Watching your favorite TV show.

__ Sitting on your favorite sofa.

__ Having your own private room.

__ Taking hot baths.

2. ***Now circle three of your favorite things you've checked above, but only three.***

HANDOUT 7-2

New Resident Tipsheet

Here are some simple things you can do to make a new resident's adjustment go a little more smoothly:

- Introduce yourself to the new resident
- Invite the resident for a tour through the facility.
- Introduce them to other residents.
- Introduce them to other staff.
- Get to know their family members.
- Learn some things about their life before the nursing home.
- Be sensitive to the possible confusion and upset that the resident and family may feel.

HANDOUT 7-3

Meeting the New Resident

— A ROLE PLAY —

1. THE NEW RESIDENT

Mrs. West is a 78-year-old new resident who has been falling more and more lately and becoming increasingly forgetful. Walking has become difficult and she can't do much for herself anymore. Her husband died three years ago and she continued living in their house alone, but she can't anymore. She refused offers from many family members to move in with them. She has been a housewife and mother in the same house for most of her life.

2. THE FAMILY MEMBER

Mrs. West's son, **Jordan West** is 54, a bachelor, who has had trouble keeping a steady job. He has worked odd jobs, as well as had an alcohol problem, for most of his life. Although he loves his mother, he doesn't have the resources to take care of her.

3. THE CNA

Lucy Brown has just found out about Mrs. West's arrival and has just come to meet her and her son.

HANDOUT 7-4

Causes of Psychosocial Distress

The Minimum Data Set (MDS) says there are two major causes for psychosocial distress in nursing home residents:

1. GRIEF OVER LOST STATUS OR ROLES

Usually, people come to terms with role changes as they age. Some have major difficulties in adjusting to these changed roles. Elderly people often feel a great sense of loss and sadness, when they realize they are not who they once were. For example, a man who was once a tailor now has arthritis and can barely feed himself. His inability to fulfill his old role can cause distress and even depression. A resident like this man may feel that he is not needed because he can longer fit in his old role. Or a woman who was a homemaker her whole life can no longer cook or clean in the nursing home, which makes her feel inadequate and useless.

2. RELATIONSHIP PROBLEMS

An aging person especially needs strong bonds to family and friends. As families have become more spread out and separated, this is difficult to achieve. Often, when separated from family, an older person will substitute friends and neighbors as his or her support network. These substitutes can sometimes help care for an elderly person, but many can't. Without any support system, a person will feel isolated and alone. Psychological feelings of loneliness and isolation can lead to depression, as well as physical problems. Think of a quiet resident, without any close friends, who has lost her husband and lives far from her children. All of these factors may lead to depression, as well as physical illness.

HANDOUT 7-5

Common Signs of Depression

Depression is an illness, not simply a passing sadness. Here are some of the signs to look for:

- A sullen, empty, "gray" mood
- Persistent pessimism, feeling defeated
- Loss of interest in activities formerly enjoyed
- Difficulty making decisions
- Lack of energy, and feeling slowed down
- Thoughts or talk of suicide
- Restlessness or irritability
- Loss of appetite and loss of weight
- Disturbed sleep, especially waking early in the morning
- Gloomy, unpleasant dreams

HANDOUT 7-6

Remember R.A.P.I.D.

The word RAPID can be a helpful tool for remembering the basic rights of your residents:

RESPECT. Respect is treating someone as your equal. It is taking what the person says seriously, regardless of their weakness of mind or body. Elders may be frail, but they are still adults and deserve the respect any adult deserves.

AUTONOMY. Autonomy is the basic right to control one's life through the choices one makes. As a CNA, you can protect a resident's autonomy by giving them choices. Help them build relationships with the people around them. Allow them as much control over their activities and schedule as possible. Rearrange your schedule to help give as many residents choices as you can.

PRIVACY. Many of your responsibilities with a resident involve privacy. Toileting, bathing, and some medical procedures can be very intimate acts. You should respect their privacy by keeping curtains and doors closed, as well as ensuring that no other residents are present.

Privacy also involves confidentiality. This mean not sharing information about a resident, unless other caregivers need to know it. Hallways and dining rooms are not the place to relay this information, as they violate confidentiality. It should only be shared in appropriate settings, like staff meetings, shift reports, and in-services.

INDEPENDENCE. Some independence has to be lost for a resident to enter a nursing facility. They can no longer take care of themselves or make all their own decisions. You need to try to help them hold onto some of their independence though, by allowing them to do things for themselves. Encourage them to do small tasks, even if you could do that task faster. Also, encourage them in recovery from an illness or injury.

DIGNITY. Dignity means someone's feeling of self worth and pride. A wound to one's dignity can be deep and devastating. Help residents retain their dignity, when their mind or body may be failing. Regardless of their physical or mental condition, they still deserve respect and need their dignity.

HANDOUT 7-7

QUIZ for Module 7

1. Depression is simply another way to say sadness. ❑ True ❑ False

2. You are the defender and protector of your resident's rights. ❑ True ❑ False

3. For the elderly, there are no possible treatments for depression. ❑ True ❑ False

4. The Resident Bill of Rights is just something posted in the nursing home to impress residents' families, not rules that you should follow.
   ❑ True ❑ False

5. Usually, moving into a nursing home feels like a new start for most people.
   ❑ True ❑ False

6. During a new resident's adjustment period, the family should never visit.
   ❑ True ❑ False

7. RAPID stands for Respect, Autonomy, Privacy, Independence, and Dignity.
   ❑ True ❑ False

8. If a new resident begs to go home, you should tell them that the nursing facility is now their home. ❑ True ❑ False

9. People with depression sometimes have thoughts of suicide, and some actually commit it. ❑ True ❑ False

10. Helping a resident adjust includes orienting them to their new surroundings and the new routine. ❑ True ❑ False

HANDOUT 8-1

Dementia Quiz

Check the correct answer for each statement below:

1. Dementia is only caused by Alzheimer's disease.

   ❑ TRUE ❑ FALSE

2. Alzheimer's has a cure.

   ❑ TRUE ❑ FALSE

3. Dementia is a natural part of growing old.

   ❑ TRUE ❑ FALSE

4. Alzheimer's runs in families.

   ❑ TRUE ❑ FALSE

5. New changes and challenges are good for someone with severe dementia.

   ❑ TRUE ❑ FALSE

6. People with dementia act up on purpose to bother you.

   ❑ TRUE ❑ FALSE

7. Since dementia is contagious, you can catch it from a resident.

   ❑ TRUE ❑ FALSE

HANDOUT 8-2

Dementia Defined

Dementia is a group of symptoms marked by impairment of a person's abilities to use his or her mind. This impairment is severe and interferes with daily functioning and the quality of life. Irreversible memory loss is the major sign of dementia and is almost always accompanied by a decline in other cognitive functioning, such as intellectual skills, judgement, and language. Rates of dementia increase dramatically as people age, from about 2-3% at age 65 to estimates as high as 30% among persons 85 and over. The majority of residents in nursing homes have some form of dementia.

HANDOUT 8-3

I.C.R.P.

Here is a four-step approach for dealing with the aggressive behavior of residents with dementia.

STEP 1: IDENTIFY what the resident's problem is.

Try to put yourself in the resident's place. What could be upsetting them? Why are they angry? Here are some common reasons that residents become aggressive:

- Anger at a past person or situation
- Pain
- Loneliness
- Fear of someone or something in the environment
- Boredom
- Problems with a visitor or other resident
- Confusion
- Hunger or thirst
- Over-stimulation
- Incontinence

HANDOUT 8-3 *continued*

I.C.R.P. *continued*

STEP 2: Try to CALM the resident.

First off, remember their anger is not meant personally for you. They may be angry at their state of dependence on you or their situation and take it out on you. They may be less able to deal with upsetting situations as they did in the past, and only be able to express themselves through anger.

The best way to calm an angry resident is to use a quiet, soothing voice, non-threatening body language, and to stay calm. Switch their focus to a more positive activity or subject. They are easily distracted and often redirecting attention will calm them.

Always ask yourself if YOU are the best one to calm their aggression. Maybe the resident prefers a certain person on staff and you can ask them for help. Maybe you'll need help from some other staff members, in case the person reacts violently. Never be afraid to ask for help with an angry resident.

HANDOUT 8-3 *continued*

I.C.R.P. *continued*

STEP 3: Try to RESOLVE the situation.

When you have calmed the angry resident, try to find a solution to the situation. Maybe you need to change their environment. Lower or raise the lights. Adjust the noise or music, if possible. Find out if they need to be toileted or if they are hungry or thirsty. Be reassuring and give them short, understandable directions, if necessary.

REMEMBER: If you think the angry resident is in pain, report it as soon as possible. The resident may require medical attention for an undiagnosed illness or injury.

HANDOUT 8-3 *continued*

I.C.R.P. *continued*

STEP 4: PREVENT the same problem from happening again.

The primary objective is always to stop the immediate anger, but you should also think ahead. See if this problem is a pattern and what you could do to stop that. Here are some questions to help you:

- How can you reduce stimulation in their environment?
- Can their schedule be changed to avoid the circumstances that seem to make them angry?
- Do they usually react in this way after a particular person visits?
- What can fellow staff members tell you about the particular behavior?
- Is the resident often hungry or thirsty at this time of day?
- Do other residents feel lonely or bored at the same time of day? Could you possibly bring these residents together?
- Does the resident's anger usually come after a specific activity?

HANDOUT 8-4

QUIZ for Module 8

1. When a resident tries to leave, because they believe they have to be somewhere, you should tell them they're wrong. ❑ True ❑ False

2. There is never a purpose to wandering. ❑ True ❑ False

3. Residents only become aggressive when staff members ask for it.
❑ True ❑ False

4. Bathing, feeding, and dressing can cause a resident to act aggressively, because they feel frustrated and confused by the situation. ❑ True ❑ False

5. I.C.R.P. stands for Identify, Calm, Resolve, Prevent. ❑ True ❑ False

6. New changes and challenges are good for residents with severe dementia.
❑ True ❑ False

7. Alzheimer's disease runs in families. ❑ True ❑ False

8. Residents with dementia act up on purpose to bother you. ❑ True ❑ False

9. Dementia rates increase as people age. ❑ True ❑ False

10. Calming music can help a resident who cannot filter out unwanted noise.
❑ True ❑ False

HANDOUT 9-1

How the Family Fits In

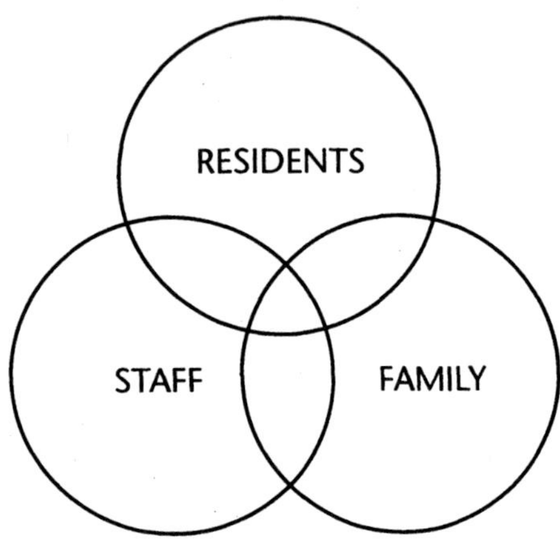

THE NURSING HOME
3 Interlocking Systems

Some people believe that you can view a nursing home as one large system made up of three smaller, interlocking systems — the residents, the staff, and the family. Because each of these three systems are interconnected, a problem in one will eventually affect the other two systems.

For instance, If there is a problem with the staff, residents and family members will both be affected by it. If there are problems among the residents, then staff and family will feel the stress, too. If family members are acting inappropriately or disagreeing with one another, then staff and residents will also feel the strain.

(Based on the work of Mary Kohl Barnwell, ACSW, quoted in *Promoting Mental Wellness in Elder Care* by Carol R. Hegeman, M.S. and Karl Pillemer, Ph.D. A publication of FLTC.)

HANDOUT 9-2

Conflict Resolution

The goal is always to walk away from conflict with a family member feeling positive about the situation. Though this can often be extremely difficult, following these five simple steps can make this process easier:

1. Have the person thoroughly explain their complaint.

2. Be clear that you understand their complaint.

3. Look for the need or reason behind the problem.

4. Come up with ideas for solutions and, by process of elimination, choose the best one.

5. Agree to a time and place to try the solution and a time to look for a new solution, if necessary.

HANDOUT 9-3

QUIZ for Module 9

1. Often, families feel guilty about placing their relative in a nursing home.
❑ True ❑ False

2. You should show the resident's family that you value their relative as an individual.
❑ True ❑ False

3. When families let CNAs know about their loved one's special needs and problems, CNAs usually provide better care. ❑ True ❑ False

4. If a family member has a care plan that is in opposition to that of the facility, you should follow theirs unquestioningly. ❑ True ❑ False

5. As the CNA, you are expected to know the answer to any question a family member might ask of you, medical or otherwise. ❑ True ❑ False

6. If there is a problem with the family, staff and residents are often affected too.
❑ True ❑ False

7. Relatives of the resident need a connection with their elder, as much as the elder needs them. ❑ True ❑ False

8. You should always try to walk away from conflict with a resident's family feeling positive about the situation. ❑ True ❑ False

9. The only solution to angry family members is to avoid them. ❑ True ❑ False

10. If family members complain unreasonably, you should look for a deeper need behind the complaint. ❑ True ❑ False

CNA
CAREER LADDER
MADE
EASY

Appendix 1: Program Forms

Career Ladder Application Form

TO BE FILLED OUT BY THE EMPLOYEE

Name: ______________________________ Job title: ____________________

Why do you want to participate in the Career Ladder Program?

____

____

____

____

____

____

____

____

____

____

I understand the rules established for the Career Ladder program for nursing assistants. I also understand that my absence from any training session associated with this program may constitute voluntary withdrawal from this program.

Employee's signature: ______________________________ Date: __________

TO BE FILLED OUT BY THE FACILITY ADMINISTRATION

Employee's date of hire: ________________ Employee's job title: ____________________

Does this employee meet our facility's eligibility requirements for this program? YES NO

I recommend this employee for participation in the Career Ladder Program:

Employee's supervisor: ______________________________ Date: __________

Director of Nursing: ______________________________ Date: __________

Administrator: ______________________________ Date: __________

Graduation Certificate — *Sample Only*

— SAMPLE ONLY —

To create your own facility's graduation certificate, use the following page and carefully photocopy it onto a blank award certificate form (using this page as your guide) found in most large stationery stores.

In recognition of the best Nursing Assistants in long-term care

does hereby confer upon

____

On this day of ______________

The title of

____

With all the honors, privileges, and responsibilities pertaining to that title.

____
ADMINISTRATOR

____
DIRECTOR OF NURSING

Graduation Certificate — *Master*

In recognition of the best Nursing Assistants in long-term care

does hereby confer upon

____

On this day of ____________________

The title of

____

With all the honors, privileges, and responsibilities pertaining to that title.

____________________ ____________________

ADMINISTRATOR DIRECTOR OF NURSING